PRAISE FOR DR. FREDERICK N. LUKASH'S *The Safe and Sane Guide to Teenage Plastic Surgery* (BenBella Books):

"…A necessary book, and one I wish had been available to the parents of the teens who underwent cosmetic procedures—200,000 of them—in the U.S. last year."

— **New Yorker.com**

"I wish this book had existed when I was seventeen years old and facing reconstructive surgery. It would have been a source of wisdom and comfort for, not just me, but my parents, too. What a Godsend this book will be for so many teens and their families."

– Jodee Blanco, **New York Times** bestselling author *Please Stop Laughing at Me*

"This book fills a definite need in public library and consumer health collections."

– **Library Journal**

PRAISE FOR THE RESTORE POINT: *The Safe and Sane Guide to A Lifetime of Lean for Kids, Teens and Families:*

"A must read for all parents and those working with children and teens! Parents today are naturally concerned with their children's intellectual, emotional and social growth, however NOT as focused on how proper nutrition is critically linked to all three. In this book, Dr. Lukash helps parents discover ways in which they can teach both themselves and their children to "take charge of their own body's destiny." Dr. Lukash carefully guides us through this journey by helping us discover our own "Restore Point." This remarkable book is both informative and pragmatic. It provides strategies to help us change our belief system regarding food. It will empower the reader to shift their cultural biases regarding their present food consumption and reframe their thoughts to enable them to "reset their child and teen's metabolism to 'The Restore Point'."

– Glenn Pollack, Ph.D., Director of the College Counseling Center at Manhattanville College; Adjunct Associate Professor, Doctoral Psychology Program, Hofstra University and Disaster Psychologist, American Red Cross.

"In this new and exciting book, Dr. Lukash brings a wealth of clinical experiences to the most important health problem of our time. He synthesizes solid, scientific evidence with his own clinical experience and outlines practical tips for the overweight teen as well as for the family who would like to start early to prevent their kids from having a weight problem. He brings the unique and valuable perspective of a pediatric plastic surgeon who has seen the effects of the obesity epidemic, firsthand. He illustrates his points with poignant stories drawn from patients who have come to him for help. I highly recommend it."

– Marc S. Jacobson, MD, Director of Pediatric Metabolic Medicine with ProHealth Care Associates and Professor of Pediatrics and Nutrition at the Albert Einstein College of Medicine.

THE RESTORE POINT

The Safe and Sane Guide to a Lifetime of Lean For Kids, Teens and Families

Frederick N. Lukash, MD, FACS, FAAP

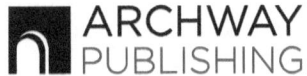

Archway Publishing books may be ordered through booksellers or by contacting:

Archway Publishing
1663 Liberty Drive
Bloomington, IN 47403
www.archwaypublishing.com
1 (888) 242-5904

Cover and interior graphics by Stephen J. Weredyk.

ISBN: 978-1-4808-1701-2 (sc)
ISBN: 978-1-4808-1702-9 (e)

Library of Congress Control Number: 2015904704

Print information available on the last page.

Archway Publishing rev. date: 4/28/2015

Dedication

*For my patients, who've taught me so much … and
for my wife and girls who continue the lessons.*

Acknowledgements

So many people have contributed to the success of this book.

First, I need to thank Long Island Plastic Surgical Group, PC, which I am proud to be a part of, for their wholehearted support and encouragement from the inception of this book to its writing and publication. The practice believes in the holistic wellness of their patients. Their 360-degree approach to patient care was a key element in their support of a book dealing with pediatric obesity—an issue affecting our patients as well as millions of individuals around the world.

Individually, I'd like to thank my editor and collaborator, Gretchen Kelly who, as always, got into my head and helped me get my thoughts on paper. Also Mark Chimsky, an editorial consultant, who helped me develop "Instinctual Wellness," the foundation for the material in this book, fifteen years ago. I need to thank Stephen Weredyk, my illustrator and designer who transformed my ideas into graphic reality. I'd also like to thank Jeanine DiGennaro, my Marketing Director and media maven who cast her always brilliant critical eye over our ideas from day one and helped bring the book to life with her fruitful contributions and encouragement.

A special "thank you" to Marc Jacobson, M.D., FAAP, FAHA, Director of Pediatric Metabolic Medicine with ProHealth Care Associates and Professor of Pediatrics and Nutrition at the Albert Einstein College of Medicine. Dr. Jacobson was an early supporter and offered invaluable critical advice on nutritional elements of the book.

Thank you, too, to Glenn Pollack, Ph.D., Director of the College

Counseling Center at Manhattanville College; Adjunct Associate Professor, Doctoral Psychology Program, Hofstra University and Disaster Psychologist, American Red Cross. Dr Pollack is a Clinical and School Psychologist, whose input into the psychological aspects of child and teen obesity have been invaluable to me through the course of writing this book, and in my practice, in general.

I'd like to acknowledge Linzy Unger, MS, RD, CDN, Clinical Nutritionist at the Hospital for Special Surgery for her insights into nutritional wellness.

Many thanks go to Harry Watnik, Certified Professional Trainer and Exercise Specialist, for allowing me to introduce readers to his innovative "Exer-Stretch" program. Watnik holds an M.A. and teaching license in Physical Education from Adelphi University. He is an authority on biomechanics and injury care and prevention and is a Member of the National and New York Athletic Trainers Association, American College of Sports Medicine and the American Running and Fitness Association. He is certified as a Strength and Conditioning Specialist and has published numerous articles on health education and fitness.

I would like to thank my kids and grandkids as well as my wife, Yaffa, for their constant support, patience and encouragement.

And finally, I would like to thank my patients who constantly give me renewed enthusiasm to move forward in my field—a field that is inherently about transformation. It is my patients' transformations—inner and outer—that never fail to inspire me.

Contents

Introduction

Why is a Plastic Surgeon Writing a "Diet" Book for Kids?

I am a father and pediatric plastic surgeon. My entire life and career is about kids.

As a father, I have watched my own children struggle with weight issues and have supported them every step of the way back to fitness.

As a pediatric plastic surgeon, I specialize in helping kids with physical anomalies find comfort and acceptance by fitting in as opposed to standing out. I only fix the things that kids can't control themselves: ears that stick out, noses that are a little too generous, under and overbites and other issues that kids are born with but that can only be changed through surgery.

But obesity is not one of these issues.

Obesity is—on many levels—a choice, and fitness is within the means of most teens and kids.

Overweight kids are suffering needlessly in our media-driven age.

I know what obese kids and teens deal with through social media bullying; as well as the face-to-face taunts and jabs that can amount to a "death by a thousand cuts" by peers and even parents and teachers.

For years now, frustrated parents have been bringing their overweight kids to my office, asking for quick-fix solutions to their obesity.

I have also followed the progress of formerly normal weight kids after infant surgery and have seen what our culture and eating patterns can do to their bodies and metabolisms.

Every time I sent a parent away, telling them their child's obesity problem could not simply be "liposucked" away or saw a formerly normal weight child packing on pounds and endangering their health and quality of life, I felt the pain of these parents and kids myself.

I decided to track the whys and wherefores of how these kids were getting fat. I also wanted to find a simple and effective solution for these families.

Working with nutritionists, exercise experts and with my own experience as a pediatric plastic surgeon, I developed a new system—The Food Wheel—that mirrors the way we naturally evolved to eat. Forget the old "Food Pyramid," I would tell parents. "Pyramids are used to bury people." A simple and effective plan for moving and eating resulted and I watched parents go away with hope in their hearts for their kids' health and happiness. The Ready Point Exercise Plan works in concert with the Restore Point for those kids needing a jump-start to physical fitness. Sneakers, jump rope, and a stretch band and you are ready to go!

"It seems so simple!" they would say.

And it is.

These parents would invariably come back months later with a child whose body had changed—taking on the contours of fitness and the glow of health—and whose outlook and hope for the future had been RESTORED and reinvigorated.

This little book of simple principles can change your child's life (and yours, too).

You and your family may have been living and eating according to ideas that are now being proved to be a quick path to a fat life. This is not your fault.

You and your kids have downloaded the equivalent of "fat malware": metabolic drags that result after eating according to culture, rather than nature.

The Restore Point Plan will do just what it says in its name—
RESTORE your families' bodies to their natural, lean, fat-burning potential.

I think it's important to state here that *The Restore Point* addresses kids, teens and family members who are dealing with issues of weight and obesity because their metabolisms are running like PCs—they have already downloaded or are in the process of downloading the fat "malware" that our society has fed them in the form of high sugar, carbohydrates, dairy and refined foods. Obviously, some kids, teens and even some adults are those lucky few that run like Macs—virtually immune to the processed food, sugar, high carb "malware" that becomes encoded into our metabolisms. These lucky few seem to be immune to gaining weight. Their lives may be more active or other factors may be at play, but it is important to note that these folks are outliers. For the majority of kids and teens and even adults—the systems described in *The Restore Point* work and work forever.

I would also like to note that *The Restore Point* is a book of principles. These are principles that will address the issue of overweight and obesity in kids, teens and adults. As a book of principles, however, it does not give you menus or shopping lists. You are free to choose your own food and eating patterns within the system.

Our food program also does not include dairy. However, dairy and the issue of dairy and children is a highly loaded issue. Culturally, Americans still view dairy as an important part of their diet—especially where children are concerned. Although our program supports a different viewpoint—one based on evolutionary food systems—we understand that for some families, the connection to dairy is too strong to eliminate. For these readers, we would suggest modifying this part of our program and reducing, rather than eliminating dairy. Low fat rather than full fat options can be chosen as well (see the section on dairy in the Food Wheel Chapter). Our book is not an all or nothing program—rather, it offers a blueprint to bring you and your family back to their Restore Point of good health and a humming, functioning metabolism.

So if you're feeling at the end of your rope, take heart. The fat is not your fault but the solution is in your hands in the form of this simple, easy-to-read and share book of principles.

Get ready to help your child RESTORE themselves to a lifetime of lean. Apply the principles to yourself and restore your own life and fitness potential.

All it takes is a turn of the page.

SECTION I

■ ■ ■

EATING

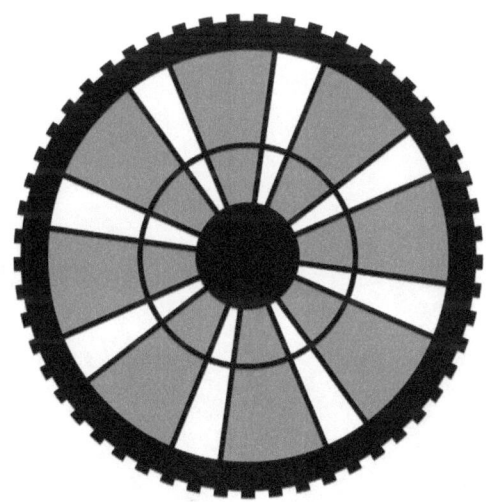

1

The Restore Point: Set Your Child Back On the Path of a Lifetime of Lean

I am a physician who specializes in pediatric and adolescent plastic surgery.

All my professional life I have seen kids and teens with physical issues who were desperately trying to just look "normal" and fit in. My first book, *The Safe and Sane Guide to Teenage Plastic Surgery* dealt in detail with these important structural problems.

In the past 15 years of my career, however, I have seen something shocking and increasingly common and avoidable: kids and teens whose state of health is more and more the tragic "norm" of obesity.

Kids and teens today are faced with a lifestyle that almost guarantees that weight problems will be part of their lives—if not now, then in the future.

Living the "virtual life" of online games and "avatars," combined with a prevalence of processed foods means that the obesity deck is stacked against kids today. In fact, this may be the first generation that lives a shorter life than their parents!

In my many years of practice, obesity-related plastic surgery was never as commonly asked for as it is today. Twenty years ago, seeing a parent who wanted a plastic surgical solution to a child's obesity was a rarity. Today, parents like these (and their obese kids and teens) fill my waiting room.

The Alarming Statistics on Childhood Obesity

(Source: National Center for Health Statistics, JAMA 2014- Prevalence of Childhood Obesity in U.S.)

- There has been a more than four-fold increase in adolescent obesity in the last 30 years
- More than one third of children and adolescents are overweight
- Three quarters of children who are clinically obese feel they are normal
- Three quarters of obese youth have at least one risk factor for heart disease
- Twenty-two percent of calories in teen diets come from sugar (CDC National Center of Health Statistics)

Sadly, many of my adolescent consultations now begin with a parent like Jessica's mom, who brings in her 17-year old for an initial appointment for liposuction. Jessica turns out to be a wonderful but frustrated teen who has suffered with several years of school bullying due to her weight.

Jessica's Story

Jessica is an example of a "perfect storm" of teenage obesity.

She's had the genetic deck stacked against her for a start. Her mother's side of the family is uniformly obese.

She's also had to deal with other major physical issues that are deeply entwined with obesity: polycystic ovary syndrome and insulin resistance.

Added to the challenges of her body makeup are behavioral issues. She's tried and failed to lose weight on both "point" and "food delivery systems."

Her family is at their wits' end and do not know how else to help her. "Can liposuction be the answer?," her mom asks me. This family is looking for the "miracle of plastic surgery" for their child. But unfortunately, the solution is not a "miracle" and Jessica is not a candidate for any kind of quick fix body contouring solution in her current obese state.

Jessica will need to undergo a life-adjustment in order for her body to change. She may even need to undergo bariatric surgery and she certainly needs to change her thinking about food and exercise. And after weight loss she probably will require multiple body contouring surgeries to restore her stretched skin to normal. (See Section III).

This is a tragedy that is far too common. And totally preventable!

We all start out at the same baseline of body wellness. Although there are large babies in nature, obesity is an acquired issue. We are not born obese. We acquire obesity through bad food habits, processed foods and lack of exercise.

Your child was born with all the internal "software" he or she needed for a lifetime of lean.

Nature gives us all we need to maintain our amazing bodies at the peak of their wellness. *We are like computers that come fresh from the factory—all our systems are working and our body "software" is fully functional and optimal.* It is through drifting away from how our bodies are meant to eat and move, that we rewire our natural fitness software and become obese. Obesity leads to inflammation, fatigue and a host of other problems that come with a fat as opposed to fit lifestyle—much as a computer acquires viruses and malware as it connects with the outside world.

Diseases of Modern Eating:

- Hypertension
- Diabetes
- Heart and vascular disease
- Gastrointestinal disorders
- Joint, muscle and skin disorders
- Psychosocial problems
- Immune disease
- Early death

The Tragedy of "Afters"

As a plastic surgeon, I am, by circumstance, at the frontlines of the pediatric obesity issue. I see the "befores" when parents bring in teens and ask me to "liposuck" their children's fat away; and I am often called in to fix the "afters"—the complicated, sometimes dangerous and always expensive issue of loose skin after massive weight loss. It is these afters—kids who had to suffer through lengthy procedures to nip and tuck their skin back into some degree of normalcy—that led me to create the **Restore Point Program**.

You may be used to seeing "magical transformations" on *The Biggest Loser* and other programs. In these shows, you start out with an obese and unhappy individual and end up with a vision of a tight and taught weight loss superstar. But the aftermath of obesity—loose skin—does not disappear with a new size 2 and a bright smile.

Samantha's story

Samantha, for instance, is a young girl in her mid-teens who comes to see me after losing close to 150 pounds on her own. She comes to my office, mom in tow, very well dressed with a bright and youthful face. But her fashionable designer clothes hide a desperate unhappiness and a secret shame. After such a large weight loss, even over the course of two years, her reward for a committed and determined effort are sagging breasts and the arms of a woman 40 years older and worse of all, loose abdominal skin that hangs to her thighs like an apron.

I begin telling Samantha and her mother that multiple surgeries will be required to re-drape and "dart" her body back to balance and proportion. These kinds of surgeries cannot be done all at once as they are too major to combine. Successive operations spaced over time including hospital stays and anesthesias are needed to give Samantha back the shape of a healthy teen. After the surgeries, there will be many incisions and permanent scars—sad reminders of an uphill battle long fought but never fully forgotten. Added to this tragedy is the cost. These procedures are not covered by most health insurance.

In addition, the time a child has to take away from school, friends and activities to undergo these operations are more factors parents need to consider. Often, a child's body image and self-esteem has been deeply damaged, and may need therapy and other support systems to become healthy again.

As a plastic surgeon, I welcome the opportunity to restore shape and contour just as I do with breast reconstruction after cancer. But if obesity and cancer could be eliminated I would happily find other problems to solve.

My goal as a physician who cares deeply about the psychosocial as well as physical development of children and teens is to stop obesity and its consequential issues *before* they begin. That is how and why I developed "**The Restore Point.**"

I have seen all too often, the aftermath of society's fat "virus" and processed food "malware" systems on our kids. I developed this program, working backward to the principles of evolutionary eating which I call, **The Restore Point**—the place that we developed from in nature **before** the historical watersheds negatively impacted our health: the agricultural revolution's introduction of grains and dairy; the industrial revolution's development of refined and processed foods and a sedentary life; and the information (or as I call it the mis-information) age where foods are marketed like travelling salesmen and "snake oil solutions," promising good health. I want our kids and parents to be at the place where our metabolism and our food options developed together to create physical bodies that function at their optimum level—the way it was intended.

The Restore Point Program can work for everyone dealing with food and weight issues; **but it is optimally used by kids and teens *before* they begin a tragic life cycle of obesity and its physical and psychological insults.**

In developing this Program, which is **not a "diet,"** but a set of easy-to-understand PRINCIPLES, I took into consideration everything I saw in the physicians' trenches of the teen and childhood obesity epidemic. Families that come to me with obese teens are at the end of their rope.

- The diet plans were too difficult, restrictive, boring, or socially debilitating.
- The gyms were too intimidating ("Everybody's body seemed to be in better shape than my own") *Our Ready Point Physical Fitness program deals with this.*
- The family lacked basic information on health and wellness and did not monitor their child's eating behavior closely.

When a parent brings a child or teen to see me because of weight problems, they usually want the quick-fix that will make them "perfect." This kind of patient is looking for a transformation from outside, not within.

A parent of an overweight teen recently said to me, "Doctor, can't you just make him look better?" But even if I changed his physical attributes, I'm not going to be able to change the core problems, which are the reasons they are *really* coming to seek help. This teen has to take charge of his own body's destiny. Then his health will improve and his feelings of desperation will be replaced by a sense of accomplishment and pride. The question is: what is he doing to help himself achieve physical and mental health? And more importantly: how is his family going to support him and join him on his quest?

Fitness – and conversely, fatness—is a family affair.

How often have you seen entire families carry the same weight problems? *If you've seen that Honey Boo-Boo reality show, you see a graphic representation of how fat is a family issue.*

If parents are obese, you will often find obese kids and teens. When kids and teens are obese, you can often find a fat or formerly fat parent.

Teens and kids don't get fat in a vacuum. Their eating habits are begun early in life.

Our End is in Our Beginning

A recent study was done by the Monell Chemical Senses Center in Philadelphia PA, on infant feeding preferences. What kids started out eating as infants is what they kept wanting as they grew. "The preferences [children] form during the first years of life actually predict what they'll eat later," Julie Mennella, a biopsychologist and researcher at the Monell Center was quoted as saying. "Dietary patterns track from early to later childhood but once they are formed, once they get older, it's really difficult to change — witness how hard it is to change the adult. You can, but it's just harder. Where you start, is where you end up."

Once kids begin school and go outside the home for food (including eating with friends in fast food restaurants), the causes of obesity are extended. By that point, many teens are carrying around a morbid amount of weight and do not even realize it since so many of their friends look and behave similarly. A recent report from the Centers from Disease Control and Prevention's National Center for Health Statistics concluded that about 30 percent of a study group of kids and teens from 8-15 years old "misperceived" their weight status (underweight, normal weight, overweight or obese). In this study, 76 percent of children and teens who were actually clinically overweight thought they were "about right." Forty-two percent of clinically obese teens perceived themselves as healthy weight and 57 percent of the obese teens and kids actually thought they were only "overweight."

The word "morbid" is used with serious forms of obesity because it can, indeed, become deadly.

I have had parents come to me thinking that if I just chisel away the fat from their child they'll find a happy, thin kid inside. It doesn't work that way. I can improve or enhance a teen or child's appearance—but for that person to be "transformed" requires inner work that only that child and their family can do together. Habits need to be changed and a new understanding of healthy patterns of eating—together as a family—need to be learned.

Mind/Body Disconnection: When the Wiring Goes Wrong

It is also important to note that you may feel you've being doing your best as a family to eat healthy and your child is still overweight. You may think, "How did this happen? I feed my kids healthy foods. They don't eat candy. What did we do wrong?"

> **Our ever-changing software is no longer compatible with our genetically fixed hard drive and operating system.**

In so many cases, the reason for obese kids and teens is not bad parenting or doing something "wrong." It is misinformation and a mind/body disconnect in a world of available processed options that cause our body's natural fueling and energy expending "software" to go awry. Our brains have outpaced our bodies.

We have created processed and refined foods that seemed progressive, but in fact have not made us healthier. They have made us sicker. You cannot be blamed for the two discordant time lines: the revolutionary brain and the evolutionary body. Again, our software has become too advanced for our PC operating systems.

A recent cover story in *National Geographic (September 2014)*, "The Evolution of Diet" explained that a hunter-gatherer food system largely dependent on healthy plants with some meat and foraged sweets is the way we have evolved to eat.

Note that this system (which mirrors The Restore Point System) is not the same as Paleo or Atkins-like programs that push meat-centric meals almost to the exclusion of natural plant-based foods.

Back to Basics- This Physician's Solution to Evolutionary Eating

In my practice, I have seen families who initially came to see me with obese kids and teens, correct their child's eating systems back to their natural, instinctual "Restore Point" using my "**Food Wheel**" system (Chapter 3) and I have seen the result: kids who can look forward to a lifetime of lean.

> **Childhood and teen years, are in fact, the best time in a person's life to reset and "restore" the natural, balanced food-to-energy system the body is meant to have.**

The Restore Point is a program based on the body's intrinsic blueprint for health. By understanding how the body has successfully functioned for millennia, you and your kids will be able to implement a lifestyle change of behavior that will help you all look your personal best, feel stronger, and glow with health both inside and out.

Small, Simple and Powerful

It is important to understand that this small book, which can be read through in an afternoon—is a powerful book of **principles** that can be learned, practiced and fused if desired to many healthy menu plans or so called "diets" in the mainstream: Atkins, Sugar Busters, South Beach, Weight Watchers, etc. **But it is not a diet—it is a plan for restoring your child's body (and your own) to a lifetime of lean—note, I said *lifetime*. This is a life plan, not a temporary fix. Once you understand it you will be freed from a library of books and programs.**

The Restore Point is a protocol that—like the computer program of the same name on a PC—will turn your teen or child's body back to its original, balanced, fat-burning, fully functional state.

> **Understand this simple principle:**
> **The software must be compatible with the operating system.**

Time and time again, I have seen kids, teens and their parents take this program, make it their own and transform their bodies and their lives—together as a family. I have seen parents who initially thought that a quick-fix surgery could change the course of their obese kids' life, adopt *The Restore Point Program* at a critical juncture in that child's life thus avoiding morbid obesity and its aftermath.

I have also personally followed this program and found new vitality and reserves of energy I never thought I'd have in my middle age. I've stayed lean and fit while many of my same-age colleagues are unsuccessfully battling their expanding guts and tightening belts.

What I'm sharing here is a program that will change your teen or child's physical destiny from fat to fit; from obese to lean—a *lifetime* of lean. Plan to set your own destiny in that direction, too and let's move forward!

2

How Obesity Went Viral:
The Restore Point and the Fat Download

I discovered the foundations for *The Restore Point* early in my career.

As a 3rd year medical student in 1971, I was accustomed to going the extra mile—trying out harmless experiments on myself based on the current lessons I was learning on various functions of the body.

Reading about metabolism in the "Bible" of medical school, the *Cecil-Loeb Textbook of Medicine*—I began learning about *gluconeogenesis* and the accompanying metabolic process, *ketosis*.

Without getting into major biological science, these two processes are about sugar and the ways that the body can maintain necessary glucose levels by burning fat. After 48 hours of losing stores of carbohydrates, metabolism kicks up to pull energy directly from stored fat so that the body can provide the needed glucose for the brain, the only fuel the brain uses.

> **When the body is depleted of sugar stores in the form of carbs, it starts drawing on fat deposits to make up for the energy loss.**

Back in 1971, there were no Atkins, or South Beach diets. Losing weight was about counting calories. A calorie was a calorie was a calorie went the thinking. As long as you limited them—no matter what they were made of—you'd lose weight.

I decided to challenge this thinking and put the theory to the test on my own body, reasoning that if I eliminated refined sugars and carbs from my diet, my body would charge up its fat burning process and through gluconeogenesis I would lose weight.

I focused on eating proteins like lean meats and fish, added a wealth of vegetables and pulpy fruits to my diet and completely—and I mean completely—eliminated bread, pasta, rice, pastry, cereals. No refined or processed carbohydrate sources.

Even though I was hardly overweight I lost 20 pounds in two months.

I put this exercise down to a learning experience, obtained my degrees and began my practice specializing in pediatric plastic surgery, focusing on infants.

The babies I cared for through surgeries for things like cleft palates and body anomalies soon grew up to be teenagers. Following them through their lives, touching base with them to make sure their early results did not need tweaking as they matured, I discovered something shocking.

A large number of these infants grew up to be overweight teens.

This had nothing to do with their cleft palates or other structural body issues. This had to do with what they were being fed—both by their parents and the culture they were living in.

Soon, the parents of these teens started coming in to ask me for help. Could surgery be a solution to their child's obesity? Could I just cut away the fat and make their child "normal" again?

Many of these families were health aware parents who did not necessarily allow their children to gorge on cookies or candy. Most of the teens I saw who were dealing with weight problems were not plagued with issues like binge eating or metabolic issues. The reason these kids were getting fat and staying fat was deeper. It was in the way we were eating as a culture. In 1988, our Surgeon General, C.

Everett Koop, declared a war on fat and promoted "fat free" carbohydrate-rich eating. Carb-loading was the trend. But if you weren't a marathon runner, this misinformation on the value of carbohydrates vs. fat actually made us collectively fatter!

How We Downloaded Fat Malware

If you think of the body as a working machine that evolved with all it needed to run efficiently—like a PC just out of the box—you can imagine our current epidemic of obesity as malware or as a virus that somehow got loaded into our system and began bogging down our hard drive.

How did this happen? It's evolutionary! Early humankind had few choices. We evolved by consuming available foods, as we adapted to our environment. We are the evolutionary descendants of these individuals. Their foods are our foods. They were high in water content, fiber, bulk, and protein, and low in salt and fat content. **Unfortunately, the early human diet was exactly the opposite of the intake of today's Information Age eaters.**

When we look to our distant past we see that early humans grazed on a diet that was abundant in water and rich in lean animal protein, fish, fruits and vegetables. Archeological and anthropological evidence and research on Hunter-Gatherer cultures shows us that ancient (what is now called "evolutionary") diets were made up of about 35% animal foods (high in protein and low in fat from lean, wild game) and 65% fruits and vegetables (carbs that were high in bulk and water content).

This is the diet our bodies evolved to eat instinctually. It's not a "Paleo" fad—it's a million-year-plus programming that wires our internal metabolic software to run smoothly and fitly.

Throughout history, our basic food sources have not changed: carbohydrates, proteins, and fats. All are necessary ingredients for maintaining well-being and providing internal cellular repair. Our bodies have also changed very little over time: less than 1% genetically. We are still programmed to instinctually crave the right foods to keep us healthy and lean.

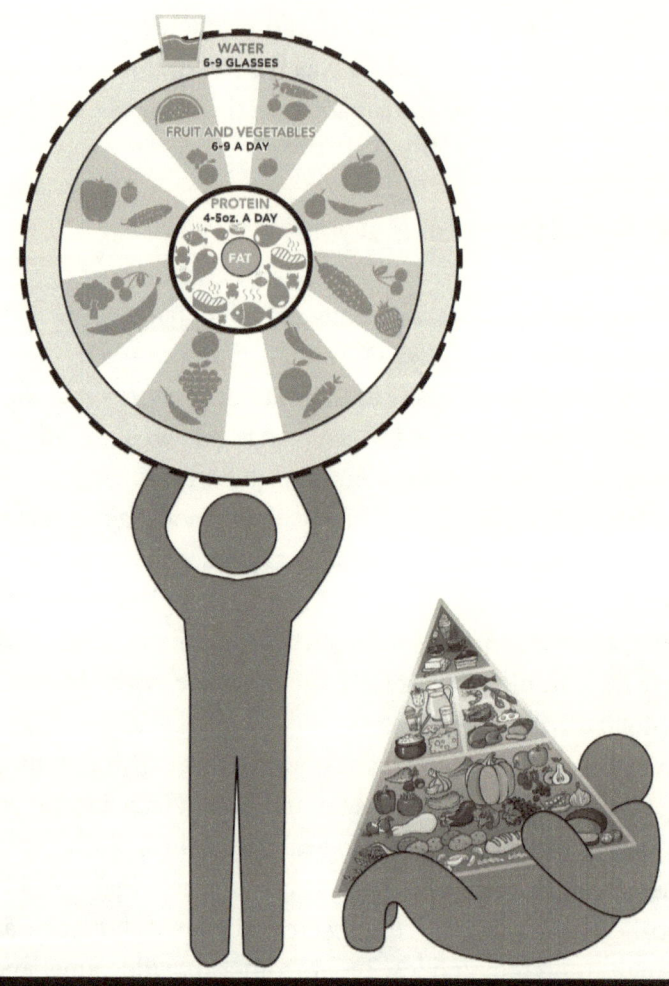

	Pre-agricultural/industrial	Avatar-information age
Protein	30% lean meat, fish, fowl	10% High fat meat
Carbohydrate	30% low glycemic fruits, vegetables	50% high glycemic grains and refined sugars
Fat	40% unsaturated fat	40% saturated fat
Fiber	High from fruits and vegetables	Low from refined foods
Water	Main source of liquid	Sugary drinks
Micronutrients	High in vitamins, antioxidants, low in salt	High free radical, high in salt

> **"Progress" has taken us away from our early instinctually correct eating patterns.**

We moved away from these naturally healthy patterns of eating lean meats when they could be found, berries, greens and other fruits to a diet dependent largely on grains and dairy products. This diet came into being during the **agricultural revolution** when grains (wheat, rice and corn) and dairy (milk, butter, cheese) became widely available.

After that came the **industrial revolution.** Railways were built that took food sources great distances to places that were not indigenous to them. Food was stored and shipped all around the world and carbohydrate-rich grains became the staple food of cattle—changing the balance of lean to fat in their meat.

Dairy was now pasteurized and the dairy industry developed around the process—marketing cow's milk as essential for healthy children and adults. Factory life set the natural grazing instinct to a time clock. Now meals were three squares a day. Milling led to further processing of foods, altering their natural states and benefits. And physical activity diminished as well. The desk job was born and bodies around the world grew more and more sedentary.

Now we are in the **Information Age** and deluged with more data about food than we know what to do with. Along with "information" comes "mis-information" in the form of media and advertising.

A recent sugared cereal commercial suggests that kids who wake up and eat a carb- and sugar-rich breakfast bowl will have energy to spare that will last the morning long, making them better students and happier kids. Another commercial for a stair-climber tells you that 15 minutes a day is all you need to get a rock-hard "six pack" of abs. An ad for white bread spins the tale that the processed slices are so rich in vitamins that you hardly need to eat anything else. Diet soda ads push low calorie sodas as a main source of hydration. Nothing wrong with swigging down soda after soda, they say, because there are no calories!

The media conveys messages like this about food, diet and exercise and we take it all in, believing the majority of tales spun from the minds of the advertising and marketing world.

Today, our information age families are inundated with choices—many, if not most of them, unhealthy. The processed and packaged food revolution is, in most cases, nothing more than viruses and malware—**processed poisons** – corrupting our operating systems – our bodies and those of our growing children.

Ancient diets were high in bulk and low in caloric density. **It took 5 pounds of that food to yield 3,000 calories. But today, with processed and packaged foods as well as "fast foods" it takes only ½ pound of such highly compact food to yield the same amount of calories.**

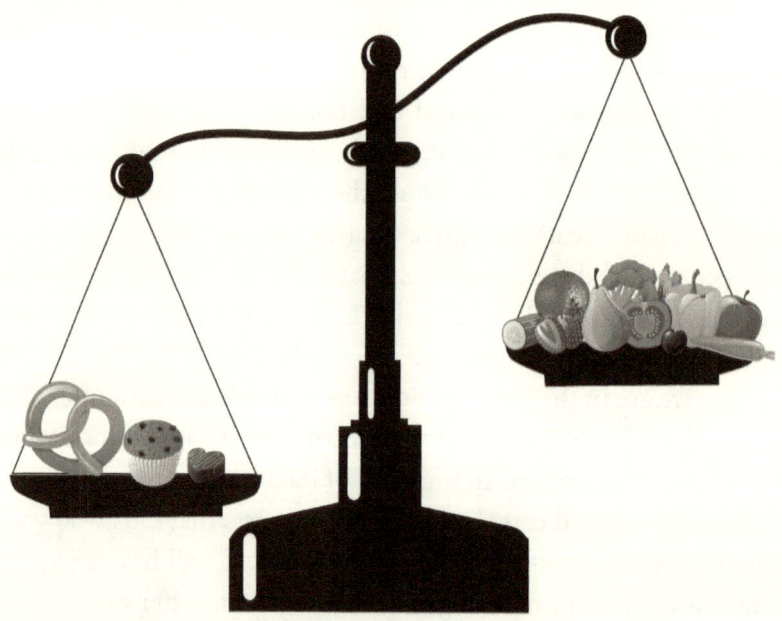

Early human consumption of sugar was rare and limited to the times when someone might stumble upon a honeycomb. Simple sugars made up less than 5% of the early human diet. **Today, American diets are made up of over 18% sugar products and the rate is increasing.**

So what's the problem today?

> Our kids' bodies are running on software that was not evolved to cope with the increased abundance and types of food we are feeding them.

Scientists and doctors have realized that accumulated body fat is not *inert*—it is an active and detrimental force that is actually aging kids and reducing ultimate life expectancy.

Historically, humans were in a famine state most of the time. Therefore, insulin (the hormone that regulates sugar metabolism) was needed to store ingested energy as fat for later use. Today, insulin is working overtime because the body is receiving sugar faster than it can be used. *All* the excess sugar is being stored as fat. However the body never gets to re-convert it because more sugar is being ingested all the time. As the body is stressed with continuous amounts of sugar the pancreas (the insulin regulator) cannot relax. It pours out insulin; forcing your blood sugar down and making you crave more glucose to bring your blood sugar level up.

This continued state of hyperinsulinism leads to increased fat deposition. Eventually, the feedback mechanism from our cells shuts down and this pancreatic hormone loses its effectiveness, leading to "insulin resistance." The pancreas now continues to pour out ineffective insulin until it fails, resulting in Type II adult onset diabetes.

"Not In My Wheelhouse"

If you and your kids eat high-fiber food, digestion is slowed and less insulin is secreted. More protein and fat and less refined carbohydrate will decrease insulin levels. If the carbohydrate sources contain high fiber, then less sugar will be released. Fructose, the sugar in fruit, will stimulate less of an insulin response than refined and processed sugar sources. As we've discussed, the body fears famine. If your kids graze all day, their bodies will feel secure. If they skip meals, their "internal food metabolising software" will panic and set itself up for starvation mode, slowing its metabolic rate and storing energy as fat for later use.

The goal of nutrition is to provide the body with nutrients without hyperinsulinism. *The Restore Point Program* helps to de-stress the body by providing it with a balance of good carbohydrate, protein, and fat for healthy living.

> **The program creates a "restore point" the way a computer does and takes the body's food processing/calorie using systems back to their original working model—the one we naturally evolved to live with as lean and healthy throughout our lives.**

"Cave Consciousness"

To set your family's own Restore Point back to working order, I want you to go back to your DNA roots as Hunter-Foragers.

Think of yourselves as now having to **hunt down** lean food sources through a forest of fat-inducing, over-processed choices, and **foraging** for food choices,whether at home or eating out, that set your body's natural fat burning systems to their original Restore Point.

As we work through the easy-to-understand principles in this book you will learn how to implement them in whatever food and menu plan suits you best.

> **What I want you to be aware of however, is eating processed foods like frozen dinners and pre-packaged goodies as well as working up elaborate "substitutes" for "bad foods" like cookies, cakes, donuts, etc. is not the same as re-setting your Restore Point. The principles are about eating simple and "pure foods" and relearning to like and appreciate them for what they do for you.**

There are a glut of books on the market now that offer all kinds of "Paleo," sugar free substitutions for traditional snack foods. The problem with these is not how they are made because if they are truly free of refined carbohydrates, they will be made of lean proteins, vegetables or fruits. There are two issues here: one is seeing food as a constant reward (snacking) and not as an energy source and the other is the elaborate preparation needed to make these food substitutes. Kids and particularly teens are on the run and cannot always rely on others to prepare their foods.

> We must change our thinking about food, not merely substitute new options into old food patterns that are part of the "malware problem."

If you have all the time in the world and want to bake some grain-free cookies as a special treat, go ahead. But keep the program as simple and as principle-based as you can and you'll be working The Restore Point process in a behavioral and nutritional balance that will reset your child and your family's metabolism and fat burning systems to their natural, living lean settings—forever and wherever.

The Key

Keeping with our analogy of your body as a computer with a basic operating system, I want you to think of your pancreas, the organ that secretes enzymes for digestion and regulates insulin for metabolism, as a key chip in your hard drive. Food is ingested and digested and the carbohydrates, protein and fats are broken down into their basic sugar, amino and fatty acids. Insulin is the broom that sweeps these breakdown products into our cells for immediate energy use or storage. Stored energy source is known as fat. The more energy provided, the more insulin demands are needed to store the excess. This worked well when food was simple and the body was set up for feast or famine. The problem today is that we are always feasting and this calorie dense abundance is pushing more and more ingested energy into body fat – never to be used because more keeps coming.

Food Made Simple

Much has been said regarding good foods and bad foods – good carbs, bad carbs; good fats, bad fats and good and bad proteins. What does this all mean? How do we differentiate? Carbs, proteins and fats are the sources for the health and body welfare.

Carbohydrates are an immediate source of energy. This is import-ant because our brain can only accept glucose as its fuel for optimal function. But it does not need *an abundance* of glucose. You can eat carbohydrates that are high in water content, high in fiber, and high in bulk: good carbs. Fruits and vegetables provide all the necessary sugar you need as well as the vitamins, minerals and antioxidants. The fiber in plant foods keeps carbohydrates healthful. These are "fill me up foods" and will satisfy your appetite without overburdening your pancreas – the insulin producer. These foods are low on the **glycemic index**, (the familiar term that indicates the rate of insulin production – the lower the index, the less insulin produced and the less storage of body fat). **These foods will reward your brain without punishing your body.**

Carbs that are calorie dense with a high glycemic index like ce-reals, breads, pastas, candy, chips increase your insulin production; they stress your body's metabolism yet fail to provide the benefits of nutrition. These should be considered bad carbs and severely, if not entirely eliminated.

Protein is a key to your body's health. It is responsible for growth and repair. Fifty percent of your body weight is protein. Proteins come from substances called amino acids. There are 22 Amino Acids or "AAs" that fulfill all our protein needs. We make all but nine, and these nine are called "essential amino acids," because we can only obtain them from food.

The best protein sources are those that include the essential AAs – these complete proteins are mostly derived from animals and fish. The benefits of eating protein are two-fold. Your body cannot store protein and sends a message to your brain to stop eating (proteins fill you up fast) and proteins stimulate secretion of a hormone called *glucagon*: the pancreas' anti-insulin.

Glucagon will mobilize your fat stores to provide your body with the necessary sugars you need for your brain and body function. While there are no truly bad proteins, there are less good ones – primarily those derived from plant sources. These are "incomplete proteins" because they lack one or more of the essential amino acids.

Vegetables used as protein sources exclusively (people on vegetarian or vegan diets) will require nutritional supplementation. While we respect those who choose to be vegan, it must be recognized that our evolution included, and our teeth were made for, carnivorous eating. Better choices may be to complement with fish, chicken, or lean meat. If these choices don't fit with your lifestyle, a non-meat source of complete protein for vegetarians is quinoa—which is actually a seed. Quinoa has a good amount of dietary fiber and it is low in fat but it is not a pure protein and it is high in carbohydrate-derived calories.

Fat, believe it or not, and in contradistinction to popular belief is something we need for our internal cellular function. There are good fats – the unsaturated ones that contain the omega-3 fatty acids that are found in many fish; and very low saturated fats found in lean meat products. Think about this as you are making your "fat choices." HDL: (high density lipoproteins) think of the H as healthy, comes from the low to unsaturated fats and deceases insulin production and can help protect against future heart disease. LDL: low density lipoproteins (think of the L as lethal) comes from highly saturated fat sources most often seen as trans-fat in margarine, baked goods, cereals. We choose lean meat to avoid the saturated fat found in grain-fed animals.

Healthy carbs, complete proteins and lean meat sources will power your body without taxing it and will lean you out and make you fit.

High glycemic carbs, incomplete proteins and fatty meats and foods with saturated fats will overburden your metabolism and make you fat and unhealthy.

The Disease of "Progress"

Some very serious diseases have been connected with diets and lifestyles associated with "progress." These diseases are not as prevalent in societies that pursue a hunter-gatherer/forager lifestyle. They include:

- Colon Cancer- linked to foods lacking in fiber and high in saturated fat
- Prostate Cancer – hyperinsulinism
- Autoimmune illness - lack of phytochemicals from vegetables and intake of dairy, grains
- Heart disease – increased dairy, fat
- Osteoporosis – lack of Vitamin C and D, lack of exercise
- Dental caries – increased sugar
- Hypertension – increase salt, saturated fat
- Diabetes – insulin resistance
- Obesity – increased insulin production, fat deposition
- Breast cancer- increased fat, increased estrogen (milk advances estrogen production in females)
- Diverticular disease-low fiber foods

Digest This

Restore Point eating means:

1. You focus on the Food Wheel (next chapter) and eliminate most if not all refined sugars and carbohydrates from your diet.

2. You focus on food that is as unprocessed as possible. Food from the ground (veggies), from the tree (fruits) and food you would have to hunt down to eat like fish, fowl and other animal meats without additives and fillers.

3. You eliminate most, if not all, dairy products from your diet and substitute alternatives if necessary.

4. You realize that water is the best and most complete drink available and drink it whenever you can.

5. You get as much exercise as you can (see Section II). Walking is our natural state—not sitting! This is why the earliest humans were called *Homo Erectus* meaning standing upright—not sitting in a lounge chair or in front of a computer becoming "Homo Sedenterus Obesis."

3

Restore Point Basics: A Lifetime of Lean with the Food Wheel

We are what we eat and we need to realize what we have been eating is making us sick

The matrix of the Restore Point is the **Food Wheel**.

That's a *wheel* not a pyramid or a plate.

The old U.S. Food and Drug Administration's "Food Pyramid" was created in 1992. It's organized on a top-down hierarchy: the foods promoted as healthy are on the base and foods they say we should eat sparsely are at the top.

The USDA has recently introduced a revised version of the pyramid called "the food plate." It attempts to simplify the same basic criteria (however with more fruits and vegetables suggested). It is an innocuous description of what to eat and also includes a standard "cup of dairy" right by the plate showing us that although the graphics may have changed, the concept is similar.

People are buried under pyramid's aren't they?

Time and time again, cutting edge nutritionists have questioned the value of the old Food Pyramid.

Fats, sweets and oils are at the top (basically forbidden but for a few servings). The second level is made up of dairy (2-3 servings a day) plus meat, poultry, fish, beans, eggs and nuts (2-3 servings daily). The next level is made up of fruits and vegetables with 3-5 servings listed as optimum. Cereal, rice and pasta—yes pasta—are at the base. Meaning the USDA recommends 6-11 servings of these daily.

The pyramid tombs of the ancient Egyptians, Aztecs, Mayans and Incas all were built by grain-based cultures, and are now extinct. Maybe they fell through "diseases of culture" related to food; such as heart disease, dental caries (a big problem plaguing the Egyptians), hypertension, diabetes, auto-immune diseases and osteoporosis.

If you and your family follow the traditional food pyramid with its emphasis on cereals, rice and pasta you will unquestionably be pushing a boulder up a mountain as you try to maintain your weight or conquer childhood or pediatric obesity. The body simply cannot process all that glucose and begin to draw on its stored fat fuels—burning and reducing them.

Some kids with a high metabolism can live on a diet like this until their 20's or even 30's, but sooner or later the sheer volume of sugars the body is forced to process from refined carbohydrates will overwhelm the system.

The malware of a carb-overload diet will bog down your natural fitness internal software and you will get fat. It's not an "if" but a "when" scenario.

The Reinvention of the Wheel

The Restore Point's fulcrum—the **Food Wheel**—is based on sound, time-tested principles that adhere to the basic nutrition "software" built into our bodies' evolution. Its principles are easy, basic and can be laid over many popular "diets" if desired but not necessary.

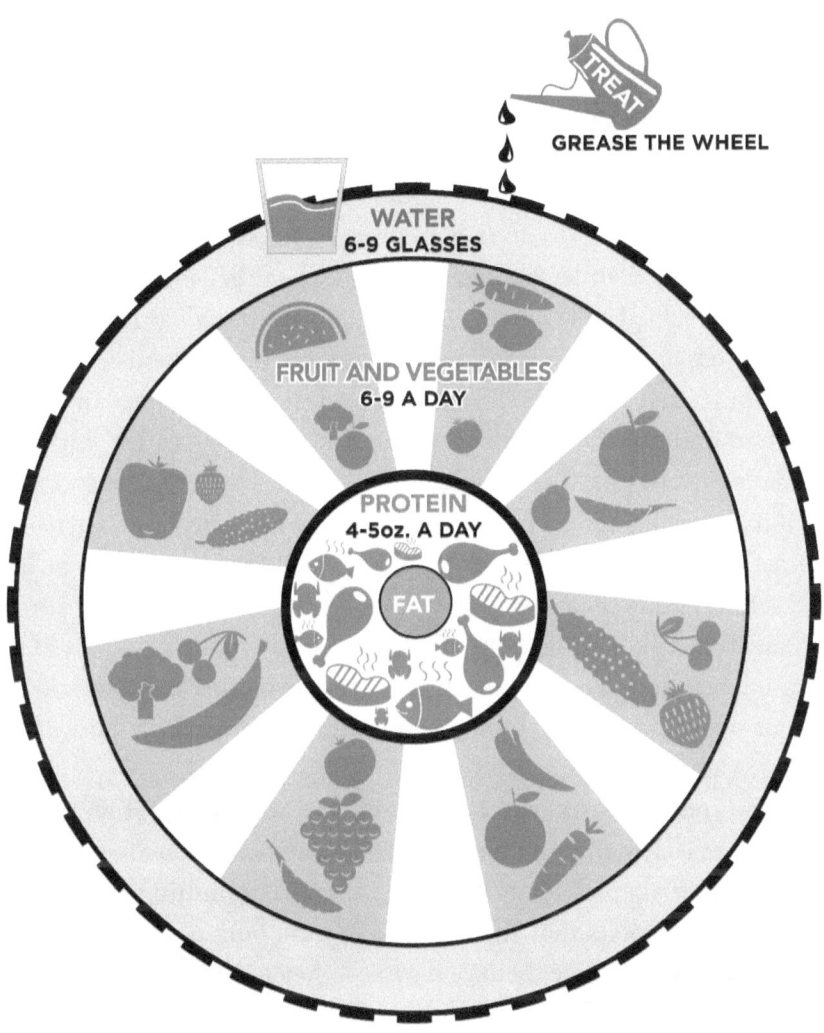

GREASE THE WHEEL

WATER
6-9 GLASSES

FRUIT AND VEGETABLES
6-9 A DAY

PROTEIN
4-5oz. A DAY

FAT

The rim of the wheel is WATER. Seventy-percent of the world is made up of water. Our bodies themselves are made up of 70 percent water. Water, it's our body's most basic HYDRATOR. **We need at least six full glasses of water a day**. Drink it often and in abundance. It's free!

When we say water, we mean water, not soda, juices, herbal teas, coffee or alcohol. Even though these liquids contain water they do not supply your body with the pure, unadulterated hydration that water does. Limit caffeinated drinks—they can create tension, encourage hunger and sleeplessness—all of which lead to overeating. Be wary of some herbal teas. Herbs are actually unregulated pharmaceuticals and can affect your child or teen's metabolism in a myriad of unexpected ways. Some herbs have even been known to affect hormones—something you don't want to do in a growing child. Read the labels on all "natural" teas to understand exactly what you're getting.

Unsweetened juices are a good alternative, especially when diluted with water to cut the caloric value. They are also a good source of vitamins C and A, and calcium. Sodas, on the other hand, can leech calcium and other nutrients from the body. Diet sodas are a whole different ball of wax. The chemicals in diet sodas have been suspected of jump-starting hunger pangs by making the body feel like it's getting something sweet (glucose) and then denying it the energy source (the sugar). The body then goes into overdrive, hyped on the anticipation of sugar energy with no pay off. Hunger is the result. So diet sodas can inadvertently make kids fat. There are also other considerations about them that are yet to be proved but are compelling. So water, water, water. And more water.

The spokes of the wheel are fruits and vegetables. High in dietary fiber, rich in micronutrients, high in water content—they are the perfect foods adapted to our body's natural programming for fitness. These are the foods that should make up the bulk of our diet—not grains, cereals and rice. Believe it or not, they are also our healthiest source of carbohydrates. Low on the glycemic index, fruits and veggies provide minimal wear and tear on our pancreas and our insulin system and therefore reduce fat deposition. They also give us essential fiber, minerals and vitamins—crucial for growing kids and teens.

Look for veggies—leafy greens, broccoli, cauliflower, spinach, asparagus, peppers, endive, arugala, kale, mesculin, rutabagas, radishes. Eat fruits like pears, apples, plums, peaches, melons, berries. These contain valuable antioxidants and fiber. The Restore Point system's Food Wheel recommends 6-9 servings of these daily—a far larger amount than the pyramid or plate does.

The hub of the wheel—and the family centerpiece of at least one meal a day—is protein. Animal protein gives us essential building blocks of amino acids. It also stimulates the pancreas to secrete glucagon, a hormone that mobilizes fat out of the body to be used as fuel. Lean meat, poultry and fish give us the complete protein our kids bodies (and our own) need on a daily basis. Poultry and fish are not only leanest sources of complete protein, they are also the lowest in saturated fat. We should eat these foods in powerful but small portions: 4-6 ounces of cooked lean meat or chicken breast per serving or 6-8 ounces of cooked fish with a maximum total of two servings per day. When fixing chicken, take off the skin and pick white meat over dark meat when you can. Avoid grain-fed beef that tends to be far fattier than grass-fed options. Avoid chopped meat where fat and carbohydrate is often used as filler.

The axel of the wheel is fat. This is at the center, the smallest portion of all the foods on the wheel. Yet, it is still critically important. Some fats like the unsaturated ones (omega-3 fatty acids) are essential for optimum health. But when it comes to fats and oils for your family, less is better. Avoid solid fats like butter and margarine (trans-fat). Ignore the health food magazines promotions of various oils like coconut and palm – stick to pure olive oil.

Olive oil is mostly monosaturated and can be used in cooking instead of butter, lard and margarine—all hydrogenated polysaturated fats. For a long time, health activists have been touting a Mediterranean diet as optimal. Scientific studies have shown that there is a lot less heart disease in countries that cook with olive oil rather than the Northern European countries that tend to cook with animal fats.

Use the small, recommended portion of fat as a condiment to accentuate your meals and make them tasty. Fat does impart flavor. Salad dressings and sauces—both used sparingly—will be all the additional fat your body needs.

Now to keep your family's bodies moving forward on the food wheel to fitness you may need to grease the wheel, not often, but periodically.

Grease represents the treats you can eat on special occasions. These are foods we may think of as forbidden temptation that make us cheat on our "diets." The Restore Point, however, is not a diet, it is a lifestyle. As part of this lifestyle a healthy amount of minor indulgence, if needed, will help keep us on the path to fitness. This may be a glass of wine for you, a small sweet treat for your child, a slice of thin-crust pizza for your teen.

That's it. That's the system. Simple, elegant and easy.

Why is it so much better for our bodies and why does it set our internal software back to its original Restore Point?

First, we exchange stimulant drinks like soda and coffee that pump us full of sugar and caffeine, for water. Pure water will keep us hydrated and help digestion, while helping us feel full and satisfied. Many times a hunger pang can be quelled with a big drink of water. Many cultures swear by plain warm water as a digestive aid.

Secondly, we eliminate refined carbs (grains, cereals, pasta, cakes, breads) that have zero bulk benefit and are incredibly high in calories and very low in nutrients. We replace them with carbs that are nutrient-rich in vitamins and minerals and are bursting with anti-oxidants—pulpy fruits and vegetables. This one, simple substitution moves the body back to its Restore Point in a powerful way. It shuts down the insulin drive to store excess sugar as fat. Unrefined oat bran (soluble fiber) and wheat bran (insoluble fiber) are the only acceptable grains to eat, along with quinoa—if you feel that you or your kids can't live without them. These are very slow digesting and low on the glycemic index. They are the most basic of carbs from the dawn of agriculture, before the advent of milling.

Thirdly, we are now centralizing our meals on a protein source, preferably lean animal meat or fish to benefit from a complete source of bodybuilding amino acids. There's a reason body builders bulk up on proteins—because it builds muscle. Vegetable protein, although healthy, does not give us the full complement of essential amino acids we need and therefore requires supplementation.

Protein from grains comes with a load of "malware" like refined carbohydrates and saturated fat. We want our protein to be lean, low in salt and low in saturated fat. What this does is to stimulate glucagon and mobilize fat from our cells to be used as energy—fat burning!

Finally, our family's fat intake should not include hydrogenated saturated fats like margarine and butter and fatty domesticated beef. Moving to lean, free-range meats and low mercury fish sources will decrease saturated fat and provide us with the healthy unsaturated fat and fatty acids needed for body repair mechanisms in both kids and parents. Our diets should contain the omega-3 fatty acids found in foods like salmon, mackerel and cod.

Nuts, a staple on health food shelves, are high in fat. Stay away from macadamia and coconut (both high in saturated fat). Avoid peanuts—they are in fact legumes and very allergenic. Many kids and teens have recently developed allergies to peanuts or have had them since birth—another reason to stay away. Peanut butter and peanut products are also high in fat and are usually salted to an extreme.

Nuts allowed include almonds and hazelnuts—both low in saturated fat with a good polyunsaturated fat to saturated fat ratio. They can be eaten in moderation regularly—a handful used as a snack. Walnuts, pecans, and sunflower seeds can also be eaten as special treats.

The Diary Dilemma—Do We Need It?

Mother's milk is the complete natural food source, genetically meant to kick-start our internal software and get us going on a lifetime of healthy living. But unlike our pre-agricultural ancestors, once we've gotten our babies off of breast milk we substitute it with other sources of dairy. We are the only species that regularly and voluntarily drinks another species' milk. Some of us have adapted, but lactose intolerance and allergies have developed in many groups of people around the world. **Although milk products do contain benefits like calcium and vitamin D, they are also high in sugar, saturated fat and cholesterol and represent a foreign protein introduced early in life, possibly setting up immune consequences later.**

Pre-agricultural people didn't have dairy and they thrived. The Restore Point Food Wheel therefore recommends that if dairy is used, it is used sparingly. Avoid whole milk, butter, cream, cheese, ice cream and sour cream. If you must eat dairy, use skim products and keep dairy low-fat. Many of the health benefits of milk are obtainable from other foods: for example, you can get calcium from fortified juices and leafy green vegetables. Think about milk alternatives like unsweetened almond milk and unsweetened hemp milk.

Other issues regarding dairy products include where the dairy source comes from. There are a great many studies that point to commercially sold milk as a source of unwanted antibiotics and other additives. Organic milk sources resolve some of these issues, but the questions remain: when you drink milk or eat milk/dairy products like yogurt, ice cream, cheese, butter, fermented milk products, sour crème what are you taking in?

If your food family life includes cultural connections to milk and milk products that are too strong to modify, we recommend the following:

- Choose organic milk products if you can afford them (they are usually more expensive than non-organic products).
- Choose low fat versions of the milk products you use.
- Use milk products in MODERATION. Do not rely on milk as a "growth food" or a vitamin supplement for vitamin D or Calcium.

Eggs were (and are) a mainstay of pre-agricultural societies, although once were thought of as a delicacy because of limited supply. Egg whites are pure protein and can be eaten as protein sources regularly. Enjoy the yolks (fat and cholesterol sources) as an occasional treat.

Try to eat fresh food as opposed to canned foods and frozen foods that can be packaged with sugar or salt. Check labels to look for sugar, salt, and other additives. **The most important step in re-setting your teen or child's Restore Point to its original healthy optimum is to** eliminate processed, baked and fried foods such as cookies, candy, pretzels, cakes, breads and muffins from your family's diet. These foods are energy-dense (highly caloric), low in bulk, high in refined carbohydrate and high in saturated fat. Eating them results in "failure to fill"—meaning we don't feel sated and crave more, causing an overload to our systems much as when a computer downloads a virus and starts processing slowly. The resultant fat storage and metabolism problems put the body back into pre-Restore Point damage. Don't eat them. Don't let your kids eat them.

Fallacious Food Faith vs. Restore Point Science

Isn't pasta and pizza America's favorite meal? What about all those healthy, active kids running and jumping and then relaxing with a candy bar—how bad can that be? Aren't sweets and sugar a part of a normal kid's childhood?

In order to help reset your child or teen's metabolism to their Restore Point (and your own, too, for that matter) it is imperative that we accept the fact that many of our long cherished beliefs about food are wrong. They are *culturally* designed as opposed to being *genetically generated*. Once, you as a family agree to change your belief systems, rather than constantly negotiating with them you can begin to effect real, healthy progress—resetting your family's Restore Point for a lifetime.

Reward or Punish

We need to eat according to our genetic needs almost all the time—with occasional treats as rewards for following the Food Wheel. This is the opposite of how we are used to dealing with food. Most of us eat poorly most of the time and then punish ourselves with the negative challenge of a "diet." Diets never work because the whole process is negative. It's like holding your breath. Eventually you exhale - and cheat. This further lowers self-esteem because once again you've failed.

The Restore Point Program teaches you and your family that it's not a diet or a deviation from normal eating—it *is* normal eating. It is the way nature and evolution designed our bodies to function optimally. **It's the equivalent of a clean computer, with optimal and effective internal software that helps us do what we want to do, go where we want to go and live the way we want to live in a body that's lean, attractive and above all, healthy.**

That's a gift to give to your teen or child that will last him or her a lifetime. And a gift to give yourself, too.

Digest This

Pressure points: Do These Circumstances Make You or Your Kids Want to Eat?

- Peer pressure – fast foods, social outings, "life on the go"
- Food traps at home- family not on board with program – pantry and refrigerator filled with food challenges
- Seasonal and event challenges (ice cream in the summer, heavier foods in the winter, candy at holidays and parties)
- A trip to the supermarket where bad foods are right in the center and make you impulse-buy
- Eating out (waiters pushing desert specials, bread on table, etc.)

Say "No" to Pressure Points: "First you make your work plan and then you make your plan work." Know what you will and will not eat as you go through each day and view events as challenges that you will overcome.

4

Setting Your Family's Personal Restore Point

Now that you know all about the Food Wheel—the centerpiece of the Restore Point Plan—you also now know that you haven't been deliberately doing anything wrong, **you've just been using wrong information.**

You've been accustomed to thinking that eating "fat free" including an abundance of refined carbohydrate was the best way. After all, there was a time when even our Surgeon General was promoting that thinking! If these dense food stuffs were within caloric limits, then your teen or child would not be dealing with overweight and possibly obesity.

If you have accepted popular wisdom—the traditional food pyramid—you've been using data that is inherently going to load your child's metabolism with fat-producing malware.

But with the proper program—The Restore Point Food Wheel— you now know you can reset your child's metabolism while he or she is still young, the best time to change habits and to get fit and stay fit for the rest of their lives.

Now we're going to talk about ways to incorporate the Food Wheel into your everyday life. First, lets look at how you and your family— including your overweight child or teen—are eating now. Put aside guilt or preconceptions and look at the questions below:

1. What foods do you and your family share as family meals? Pizza, pasta? Chicken, beef, fish? Do vegetables play a central part on your meal table? Do you eat as a family? Do you eat the same things? Do you eat out often and allow random menu choices because it is simple and less stressful? *Nutrition and health are <u>team efforts</u>. Meals should be discussed and planned. If going out, make a game plan. Go on line and download the menu and organize your meal.*

2. What foods do you currently put on a "forbidden list" for your kids. Why? Do you have two standards – one for you and one for your kids? *Again, there cannot be a double standard. "Do what I say and not what I do," doesn't work with families and fitness.*

3. Do processed foods or convenience foods play a central part in your home eating life? Do you follow the same healthy rules when eating out? *The* Food Wheel *gives you a set of principles to carry forward wherever you are—even in restaurants and others' homes. <u>It reminds you what to eat and what not to eat.</u>*

4. Does your overweight child or teen have any specific food cravings? Sugar? Carbs? Why is this? Is it social? Cultural? *List them with your child. Admit your food flaws and work together to purify and simplify your eating. Make it a <u>team effort</u> and don't let your child feel ostracized or isolated.*

5. Is there a specific time of day that you find them snacking or binge eating? Does it relate to boredom? Is there too much sedentary time where eating is an activity as opposed to organized exercise where food is replenishment fuel? *We eat to live not live to eat. <u>Food is not a substitute activity</u>.*

6. Do you have an ethnic or family-based food tradition that you follow? Is it set in stone? Can it be modified? *Look for ways to modify your traditions with healthy alternatives. Reduce portions of those foods which are culturally essential but not in the essential part of the food wheel.*

7. Who does your food shopping? *This can be a great training exercise for children and especially teens soon to go off on their own to learn how to "hunt and gather" in the markets. Teach them that the perimeter is where the healthy food is and the center of the market is where you find the least healthy although psychologically desirable- comfort foods.*

8. Do you and your spouse drink alcohol in the home? After dinner? Before dinner? *These are empty calories that create image problems for kids that will carry over when they go off to college and make their own choices based on imprinted behaviors. Teach the older kids about the caloric challenges of alcohol and the appetite stimulation that goes along with social drinking.*

9. Have you ever put your teen or child on a restrictive diet? Was this anxiety provoking? Did it set up negative communication barriers? Did it alienate the overweight child from his/her siblings that may not be faced with weight issues and dietary restrictions. *Never speak in terms of dieting. What are the first three letters -"D.I.E."- so negative. Speak in terms of long-term health and well-being. Look to protect the future and have a long and healthy life. Discuss the illnesses that are factually linked to unhealthy eating.*

The key to the Restore Point Nutrition Plan is **simplicity.** You'll be surprised how easy this program is once you commit to it. You'll find you will all feel better and look better—and you'll be able to be more active than you ever thought you could be!

> Our ancient past provides us with every clue we need of how we were designed to eat.
>
> We need to:
>
> 1. **Reduce total fat and look for unsaturated sources**
> 2. **Reduce salt**
> 3. **Increase fiber**
> 4. **Create a balanced diet of 60% carbohydrates, 20% protein, and 20% fat—the right kinds**
> 5. **Drink an abundance of fresh, pure water**

Phasing In the Restore Point Program: Dilution is the Solution to Pollution

Some of you may want to dive right in to the Restore Point way of eating. You may want to "clean your body out" by starting to follow the Food Wheel immediately. Others may want or need a more gradual, phased eating program. In order to manage your menus effectively you can cut out the "toxic foods" from your body in stages.

For example: In Week 1, you'll increase your intake of water. In Week 2, you'll cut out fatty red meats from your diet and incorporate fish, free-range chicken or grass fed beef. In Week 3, you'll begin to cut down on the grains you consume: whole-grain bread at only one meal per day and no cereal at all. In Week 4, you'll completely cut out all grains (no bread with any meal) and you'll treat yourself to only one non-fruit dessert for the whole week. **A tip for smart weight loss is to graze on the "fill me up foods" like fruits and veggies and not always be pigeonholed into three square meals a day. This keeps your metabolic engine purring all the time.**

My program utilizes the "eat/treat" cycle so that you avoid the "cheat/repeat" cycle of yo-yo dieting. I don't want you to feel deprived. We still have to live and not just exist. If you've maintained your family on the plan, you all deserve an occasional reward. I really love chocolate. When I go out with my wife on a Saturday night, I might order a small desert to treat myself for sticking to the Food Wheel all through the week. I know I'm not going to have this kind of dessert every night, so it becomes extra special. Because I'm in control of my nutrition, I'm also in control of when I can reward myself. Many will find that these so called rewards are not necessary and even worrisome; that they might re-trigger the need for the unhealthy. When I am challenged I order fruit for dessert and put the worry behind me.

When our Hunter-Gatherer ancestors chanced upon a beehive, they recognized the honey within was sweet and so they lapped it up. They didn't know when they would discover the next beehive, so they made the most of their unexpected "dessert." Culturally, we know when we can have the next treat because we choose when we're going to reward ourselves. We are in control of what we eat and when we eat it. We need to exercise that control!

Freedom and Flexibility

Different approaches appeal to different people and the Restore Point eating program has a variety of menus to choose from. There is room for a wide range of variations on the theme of the basics (chicken, lean meat, fish, fruit, and vegetables). The Food Wheel lets you interchange these basics to your own particular taste and habits. That's part of the ease and flexibility of the program.

Remember this is a life plan. If you fall off the wheel – get back on.

Eating Out

When dining out, you may sometimes need to make requests—substituting vegetables for pasta, for example—but you should have no trouble applying the food wheel roadmap to any situation. If you know where you are going you can look at the menu on-line and even call in advance to see if they will accommodate your choices.

How to Read a Menu

Eating out doesn't have to mean restricting yourself to salads with no dressing. Believe it or not you can go out with friends and family and stay **RESTORE POINT-ready**

Here are some basic principles:

1. **Consider asking for the gluten-free menu.** Many restaurants are now doing gluten-free menus for the millions of Americans who are demanding them. Gluten-free means wheat-free so this will basically be a bread-free menu. Watch out for potatoes and rice. You'll find gluten-free menus may give you more FOOD WHEEL FRIENDLY options than you realize. Important to note though that gluten-free does not automatically mean healthier. Some store-bought gluten-free products are more highly processed and high in calories and sugar. Check out potential gluten-free menu options but *caveat emptor*, let the buyer beware, and if you're unsure of a dish, go with more familiar choices on the food wheel.

2. **Check side dishes first.** This is where veggies in various forms often live. A side dish of spinach or zucchini is often a great choice in Italian restaurants. Chinese restaurants often have steamed vegetables listed here. Mexican restaurants have nice salads with avocado (good fat). Order fajitas and leave off the tacos and you have protein and vegetables. Greek restaurants are ready made for us with salads, fish and vegetables.

3. **Ask for food without MSG.** It's a filling agent containing chemicals you don't need in your body. And you'll be hungrier later if you are filled up on MSG now.

4. **Salads can be main dishes.** Restaurants are also usually amenable to custom-designing your salad: dressing on the side is the best way to go with olive oil and balsamic vinegar and lemon or a light vinaigrette. Add a protein like chicken, steak, tuna or shrimp.

5. **Choose fresh fruit for dessert.** It is filling, refreshing and you are not socially isolating yourself.

6. **Even fast food places have what you need if you "hunt and forage."** Salad bars, fruits, and protein dishes – get rid of the bread. Look for grilled rather than fried meat or fish.

7. **Ask the waiter to remove the bread and bring a vegetable dish.**

8. **Actually drink the water placed on your table** – it will begin to satiate you and not drive appetite like soda or alcohol will.

9. **Social eating is part of our culture but must involve thinking and not mindless ingestion.**

10. **Avoid those "shared deserts"** – the big one in the center with all the spoons – you will eat more than you think – and regret it later.

The Restore Point Field Guide to Fast Food

I have done extensive investigation in the major fast food chains and discovered there are healthy dishes to order in each one of them.

So, if McDonald's, Taco Bell, Burger King, KFC or Wendy's is your only family option, don't despair: there *will be* meals you can eat that will be part of the program.

The dynamic to work here is your hunter/gatherer ancestors'— think HUNTING for healthy food options when eating out.

Hunt for clean protein options like grilled chicken, lean beef (no special sauce). Side salads are offered in almost all fast food chains. You can order a grilled chicken sandwich or burrito and take it out of its grain/carb pouch and mix onto a side salad for an inexpensive and totally FOOD WHEEL FRIENDLY meal.

Beverages include tap water (cheap and plentiful!), seltzer, unsweetened ice tea and black coffee. Limit the dairy to skim or fat free milk and if you use sugar substitutes – do it sparingly.

McDonalds:

Side salads, grilled chicken, fruit cup, Egg McMuffin without the Muffin (McDonald's is now also offering a new Egg White Egg McMuffin, which you can have as long as you don't eat the muffin).

KFC:

Grilled chicken options (remove the skin).

Wendy's:

Main course salads, grilled chicken sandwiches (leave off bread), scooped out baked potatoes (if all else fails) – eat the skins.

Chinese Take Out:

Steamed vegetables with chicken, beef or seafood. Stay away from tofu—as a surgeon, I'm concerned about hormone issues in soy foods.

Mexican/Taco Bell

Beef or chicken tacos minus the taco on a salad bed. Avocado is a healthy fat.

The Truth About Supplements for Kids, Teens and Adults, Too

Too often people are under the impression that we need a home pharmacy of supplements because our diet is lacking in them. Since we live in the midst of an abundance of foods, we can *always* find those that are rich in vitamins and minerals. We do not need to load up on pills, when the micronutrients we need are already in the foods we eat. A multivitamin is not usually dangerous, but taking too many supplements is foolish, unnecessary, and could, in fact, be harmful. Supplements have become a booming industry because of poor eating choices. If you follow the Restore Point nutrition plan, you won't need vitamin supplements—you'll already be getting all the vitamins you need *naturally* in the foods you'll be eating. **Complement with healthy foods, rather than *supplement* with pills.**

The yearly physician check up will serve as a barometer of how you and your child's nutrition is working. Obviously, if there is a true deficiency then supplementation is a replacement for something actually needed. Conversely, if you are eating well and balanced, then supplements are superfluous.

Food Habits

Family   Teen

SECTION II

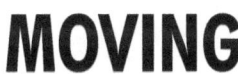

MOVING

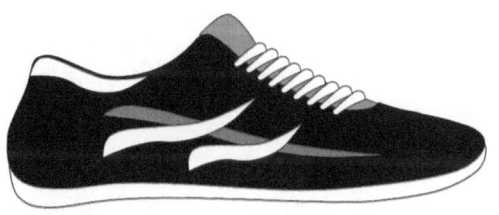

5

The Ready Point Plan for Forever Fitness: Movement, Muscle and the Power of Resistance

Now that you and your child or teen understand the "Restore Point," we are going to talk about the **"Ready Point."**

A "lifetime of lean" does not happen through food changes alone. As we all know, body wellness MUST include physical activity—especially for an overweight child or teen, and is critical to success.

It took hundreds of thousands of years to evolve into *Homo sapiens*. Throughout those eras, humans became more upright and more determined to develop physically and mentally. Since the agricultural and industrial revolutions, we seem to be regressing physically. It's as if the more technologically advanced we become, the less *"Homo sapien sapien"* we are, and the more *"**Homo sedentarius obesus**"* we are.

Even though we have servo-tools and vehicles to make our lives easier, they may not be making us live longer and healthier. Like it or not, we are genetically linked to our ancient past both nutritionally, and by our patterns of physical activity. Our body's "operator's manual" has not been programmed for sudden change. **We require both endurance and strength exercise for peak health and wellness.**

Ancient Links to Modern Fitness

The life of the Hunter-Gatherer was physically taxing, requiring stamina for the days of nomadic tracking of animals. Killing animals and lugging them back to their camps sometimes demanded Herculean strength and enormous endurance. Similarly, gathering wild fruits and vegetables required intense labor. However, research has shown that Early Man called upon such physical efforts only episodically; he could rest when there was plenty and needed to hunt and gather only when "the table was bare." From this, we get the ideal form of workout, utilizing aerobic movement, and resistance exercises to build strength. We must try to use our bodies as they were originally meant to be used: **engaging in short bursts of intense physical activity, with rest periods in between. This dynamic—also called interval training—will result in peak wellness.**

What is the best way to begin to exercise? In collaboration with a personal trainer and fitness expert, we have assembled a workout program designed to get kids, teens and families to THE READY POINT of fitness. The program alternates endurance or cardio- respiratory fitness with strength training.

Why do we call it THE READY POINT? Because when you use the program below you, and your kids and teens will find that it will get your bodies READY for life and fitness activities. Maybe your child is reluctant to participate in gym, or go to camp, for fear of athletic limitations, because of physical inactivity and obesity. We are here to get them ready for more – to jump - start them into wanting more! And it is beneficial for parents as well – and something you can do together.

What does this mean? Our exercises will maximize each area of the body while allowing for periods of recovery; it will also prevent physical breakdown and boredom from mindless repetition of routine. Workouts can be completed between 10 - 20 minutes. (How many times have you seen people spending hours on treadmills and Stairmasters, breaking down their tissues instead of building them up?) Using minimal equipment—your own body, a pair of sneakers and exercise bands and a jump rope, which you can purchase at nominal cost—you'll be able to follow a simple program of aerobic and resistance exercises that will help tone you up and build endurance as you lose weight. Resistance strength building will increase the size of the body's fat-burning engine.

Resistance is determined by how far the band is stretched between your hands or between your hand and foot. Muscle weighs more than fat, but occupies one-fifth the space. Our Fitness Formula will strengthen bones, joints, ligaments, and tendons, and build muscle, which in turn burns fat.

Other exercises that are part of the Fitness Formula workout are speed walking, jumping rope, push-ups and sit-ups. Real step climbing is an excellent way to develop the leg muscles. This aerobic exercise can be made more physically demanding by increasing the speed and number of flights of steps you climb.

Our program of Ready Point exercise will:

1. **Create the demand for increased fuel consumption.**
2. **Increase muscle mass, which will, in turn, increase fuel consumption demands.**
3. **Provide an aerobic workout for cardio-pulmonary fitness (but don't overdo or you'll wear down your joints).**
4. **Offer short, intense workouts that will stimulate muscle definition.**
5. **Produce endorphins and promote serotonin release, which is calming and satisfying.**

You'll be able to take the tools of your Fitness Formula exercise program with you anywhere: put your stretch bands and jump rope inside your sneakers and into a bag and you have your instant "mobile gym."

You can customize a workout routine that works for you anyplace you are.

Total wellness requires a blend of smart nutrition and steady exercise. Dieting alone will result in the loss of lean tissue—bone and muscle mass as well as fat. Aerobics alone will wear down joints and limit overall fitness. However, combine nutrition and aerobic and strength exercises together and you'll keep your family in maximum shape. Let's not begin the process of degeneration earlier than we are genetically and evolutionarily programmed to. We cannot go back into the wild, but let's at least get out of our "cages."

With our workout program, you can progress to jogging and running, add cycling, and swimming. All are all beneficial and can be initiated at a beginner's pace and incrementally increased to obtain maximum benefit to the heart and lungs. This will also increase the metabolic rate to burn more energy (calories) and promote weight loss. The combination of strength and endurance exercises will help you look better and feel better.

The Ready Point will put into evolutionary perspective the type of physical exertion that kids need to be healthy.

It is my belief that people who suffer from low self-esteem due to physical "un-fitness" **can turn their lives around by beginning to follow their own genetic blueprint for wellness.** Once a person feels empowered and motivated to exercise regularly, he or she can combine my program with additional activities, such as taking up an interactive sport (mine is fencing) or joining a gym. Your goal is to build up your exercise levels by degrees so that you make it part of your daily life. The Ready Point will help kids move past the fear of exercise to enjoy the joy of a lifetime of activity.

If your child or teen is visibly obese you are automatically dealing with an entire set of shame and social isolation issues that make it hard, if not impossible, for a kid to "just do it" and implement a fitness program at a gym. In fact, your child may be having major physical and psychological issues that prevent him or her from participating in social sports with other kids at the school's gym.

Obesity has many aspects and one of the most insidious ones is its power to immobilize and prevent a child or teen from getting the physical activity needed. I have personally seen this in my practice. Parents bring in their overweight child or teen and hope that a quick fix liposuction or tummy tuck will deal with some of these gym shame issues, and get their child back into life. Unfortunately, it's not that easy.

The body must be tuned like a car from the inside out. If your car isn't working properly would you take it to the garage and ask them to repaint it?

No, you would carefully and methodically figure out what mechanics were weak or faulty and repair them, step-by-step, no matter how much time it took.

That is what the READY POINT is about. Along with the RESTORE POINT nutrition plan it prepares your child's body for fitness slowly, safely and systematically building muscle, flexibility, and coordination, so that your child can get back into life.

Doctors Need Work Outs, Too

I personally found out how effective this program was when I implemented it at a time when I was being challenged in terms of my own fitness—especially around time constraints.

It may surprise you but many plastic surgeons—and a lot of physicians in general—have fitness challenges just like everyone else. Long hours in the operating room with junk food pick-me-ups and severe time constraints pose huge obstacles to regular physical exercise.

Just as I was looking for a flexible fitness solution, I met Harry Watnik, a physical trainer and exercise specialist who developed the "Exer-Stretch" program. The exercises are a comprehensive fitness solution based on resistance bands—those thick rubber stretchies you can find cheaply, in easy-to-access shops or on line.

Harry showed me how the bands in tandem with a regular cardio activity like jumping rope or climbing stairs, which could be done in my own house or in the hospital stairwells, could solve virtually all my fitness issues.

Using the bands several times a week for about 20 minutes and including 30-second intervals jumping rope, jumping jacks, or climbing stairs I soon got my body gym-style fit in a matter of months.

"Getting fit with the bands is just getting fit for life," Harry says. Everything your child does in the real world—walking to school, dancing at the prom, swimming at the beach on a summer afternoon, playing a game of soccer with friends on the weekend—all demand a certain amount of physical "readiness."

The Ready Point Plan outlined in this chapter is so flexible (just like the bands themselves!) that it can be done almost anywhere at any time of day. You can do it indoors, outdoors—even in the water for a little extra resistance.

And unlike weight training, which can put undue stress on growing muscles and bones for kids, the bands are safe and effective for all ages. They are also great fitness tools for busy adults.

I encourage you to read through the exercises in the following chapter and do them with your kids. Push through the inertia of our avatar lives—get the kids off the computer and into regular, therapeutic movement.

Do the Ready Point program with your kids 3x a week for 20 minutes tops and you will get your child's body into the state of readiness needed for a full and active life.

When your child begins to develop physical confidence and knows he or she is at that READY POINT, more options open. They will soon be able to challenge themselves in new and exciting ways that had never been available to them before.

Healthy athletic competition, group sports, dancing, hiking, skate boarding, body building—all aspects of a rich, physically active social life for a teen or child become possible at the READY POINT.

The resistance exercises outlined in the next chapter should be done in tandem with whatever cardio activity your child is able to do: jump rope (most kids can do this even for a minute), jumping jacks, jogging in place, and eventually stair climbing.

Once you and your kids feel yourself shaping up and are ready for more, begin to alternate days of Ready-Point resistance training (the full set of exercises is outlined below) with these cardio sessions (aim to increase to 30 minutes of cardio activity on alternate days). Begin to walk or jog outside.

When your child gets his or her body confidence, pick a sport they like and encourage them to practice it regularly.

The Ready Point is just the beginning of your child's lifetime of lean. Do the plan with them and get ready for a new chapter to open in your own life as well.

Digest this -Parent Point: Gym Jams—

Speak to your child's gym teacher to reduce the possibility of fat-shaming while working the program and utilize the school's athletic facilities to your child's best advantage. In fact my research has shown that many schools have adapted to alternative physical fitness programs to tailor to a child's needs. (There are before school swimming, yoga, jogging and weight training classes – serving as alternatives to the traditional group gym activities).

6

The Ready Point Program

Sneakers, stretch bands, a jump rope and you are **ready to** continue on your journey to a lifetime of lean. Our program is designed to overcome the inertia of a sedentary life and move your child and you (too) into wanting more athletically.

We start off slowly; **and please make sure that everyone is healthy enough to engage in physical activity**. The program is designed to help you not hurt you. If in doubt consult your doctor.

Below are rubber band exercises to build up muscles and aerobic exercises for increasing stamina. By alternating them you create interval training – the best way and the most evolutionary way to stay fit.

Exercise bands – we call them "Exer-Stretch" – work by resistance and tension based on how strong the bands are and where you hold them. Bands come in many different sizes and therefore degrees of difficulty in using them. Be sure to start off easy and progressively work up to maximize the benefit.

Commit to the program and you will be amazed at the changes in your body. Set aside three days a week and allow for twenty uninterrupted minutes. For extra motivation, put on music. Ancient cultures used the cadence of the drum. Whatever will drive you is what you should choose.

Having a workout buddy can also help in overcoming the desire to stay on the couch or in front of the computer. If you are a parent, make sure your child is exercising with proper form to avoid injury – bands are elastic and can snap or release.

Once again, as a first step you will begin with 10 minutes 3 times a week. As you get stronger you can increase your sets and even repeat the circuit. You can also add more aerobics on alternate days. This could be walking, jogging, swimming, cycling for 30 minutes.

Here is how the circuit works. Start with 15 seconds (and build up to 30 seconds) of jumping jacks to warm up. Next choose the band strength appropriate for your level of fitness. **Follow the diagrams below.** Tension on the band or tube increases the resistance and thus the difficulty of the exercise. It takes about 1 second per repetition therefore each set takes roughly 10 seconds. Allow for a 10 second rest and then try and repeat 1 or 2 more times if you can – if not build up to it. Now do 15 -30 seconds of another aerobics –alternating, stair climbing, shadow boxing, jogging in place, jumping rope. After completing this start the next band set. By working through the band sets and alternating the aerobics you will have approximately a 10 - 20 - minute interval workout. Add controlled sit-ups with knees bent. The core improves by keeping your shoulders back and lifting off the floor. Push -ups complete the routine and can be done on your knees in the beginning. Sit-ups and push-ups are as many as you can do in 30 seconds.

During all your exercises, you'll want to make sure that your abdominal muscles are contracted in order to support your lower back. Each time you stretch the band, breathe out. Again you'll want to do 10 stretches for each position. For the exercise session to be aerobic, your heart rate should be elevated to at least 60% and no higher than 80% of its maximum, which is the number 220, minus your age. Your heart rate will be sustained if there is no significant pause between band sets and the aerobic exercises. If you are just beginning the Ready Point fitness program, check your pulse every five minutes to help you stay within your target zone. Work harder if you are below target and back off if you are exceeding it.

Biceps

THINK FRONT UPPER ARM MUSCLES!

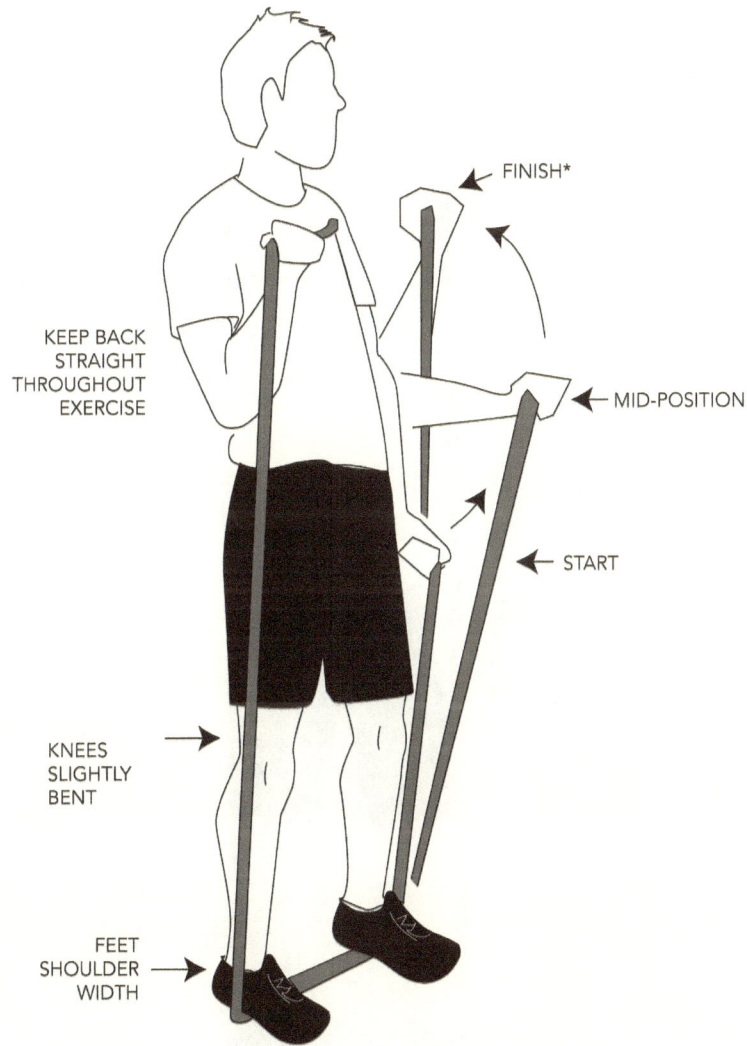

FINISH*

KEEP BACK
STRAIGHT
THROUGHOUT
EXERCISE

MID-POSITION

START

KNEES
SLIGHTLY
BENT

FEET
SHOULDER
WIDTH

*CAN DO TOGETHER OR ALTERNATE ONE ARM UP-ONE ARM DOWN

Step on the band and hold the ends in your hands. Now bend your arms at the elbow and feel your biceps respond.

Upward Press

THINK SHOULDER MUSCLES!

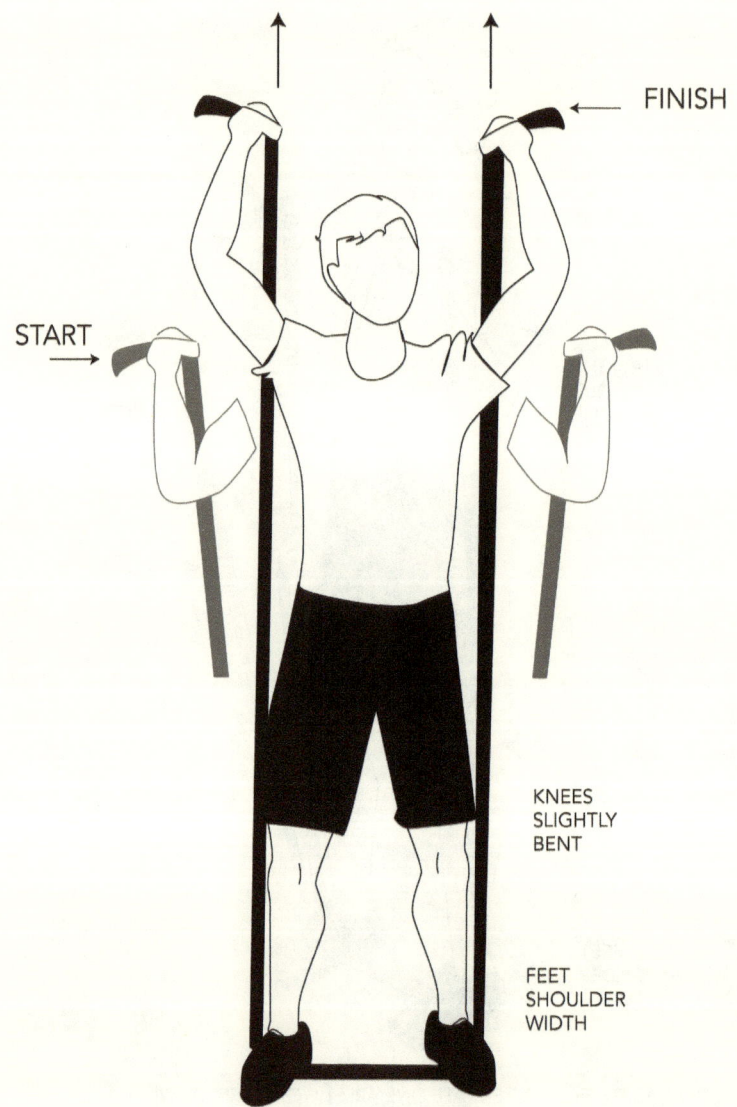

FINISH

START

KNEES
SLIGHTLY
BENT

FEET
SHOULDER
WIDTH

Step on the band and push straight up over your head with the band
behind your shoulders.

Triceps

THINK REAR UPPER ARM MUSCLES!

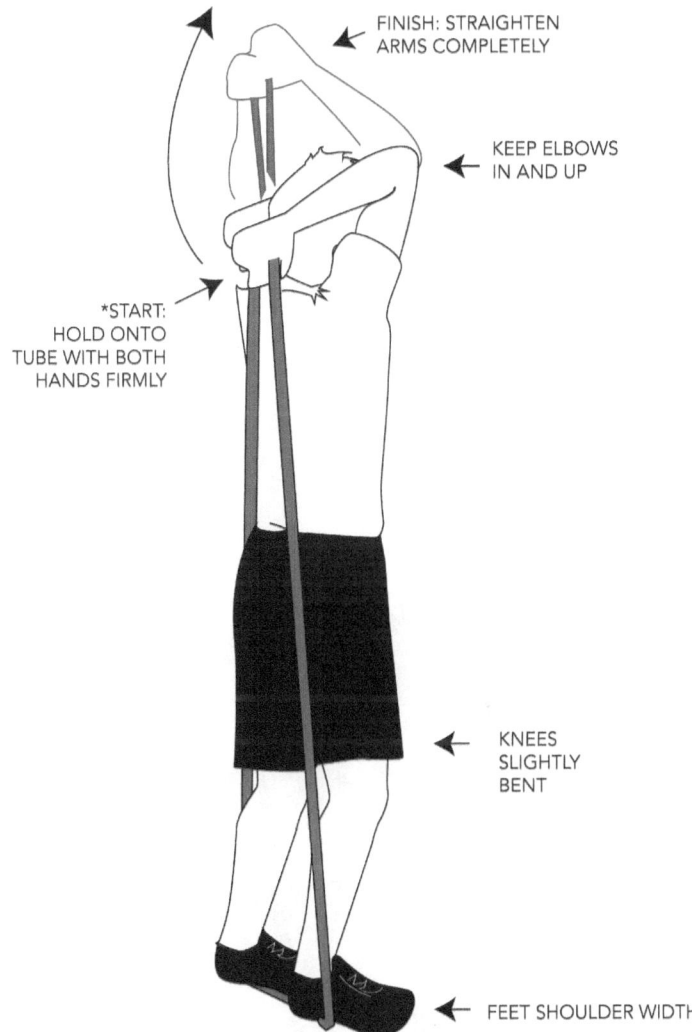

FINISH: STRAIGHTEN ARMS COMPLETELY

KEEP ELBOWS IN AND UP

*START: HOLD ONTO TUBE WITH BOTH HANDS FIRMLY

KNEES SLIGHTLY BENT

FEET SHOULDER WIDTH

* IF TOO DIFFICULT DO ONE ARM WITH ONE TUBE (WITH LESS TENSION) AT A TIME

Step on the band and grasp the ends behind your back and lift up straightening your elbows.

Quad Squats

THINK BUTTOCKS, BACK AND THIGHS!

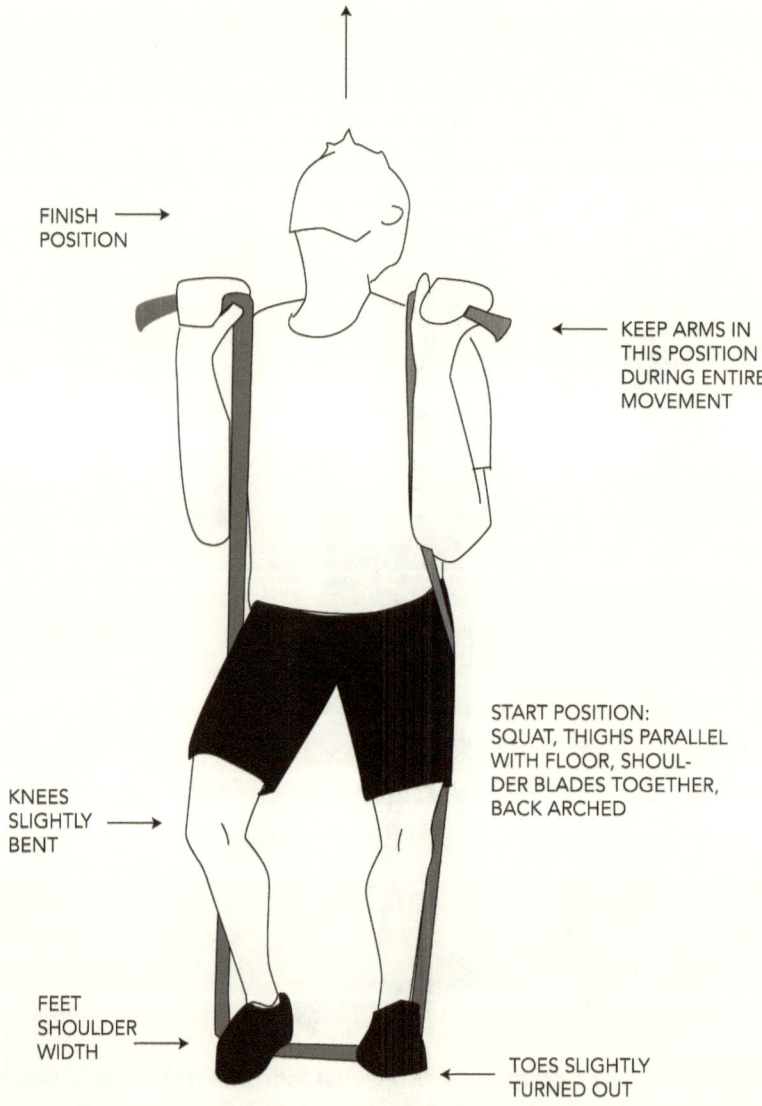

FINISH POSITION →

← KEEP ARMS IN THIS POSITION DURING ENTIRE MOVEMENT

START POSITION: SQUAT, THIGHS PARALLEL WITH FLOOR, SHOULDER BLADES TOGETHER, BACK ARCHED

KNEES SLIGHTLY BENT →

FEET SHOULDER WIDTH →

← TOES SLIGHTLY TURNED OUT

Step on the band as if you were to do a shoulder press. With tension on the band bend your knees and then push up with your legs. Repeat.

Side Core

THINK WAIST MUSCLES!

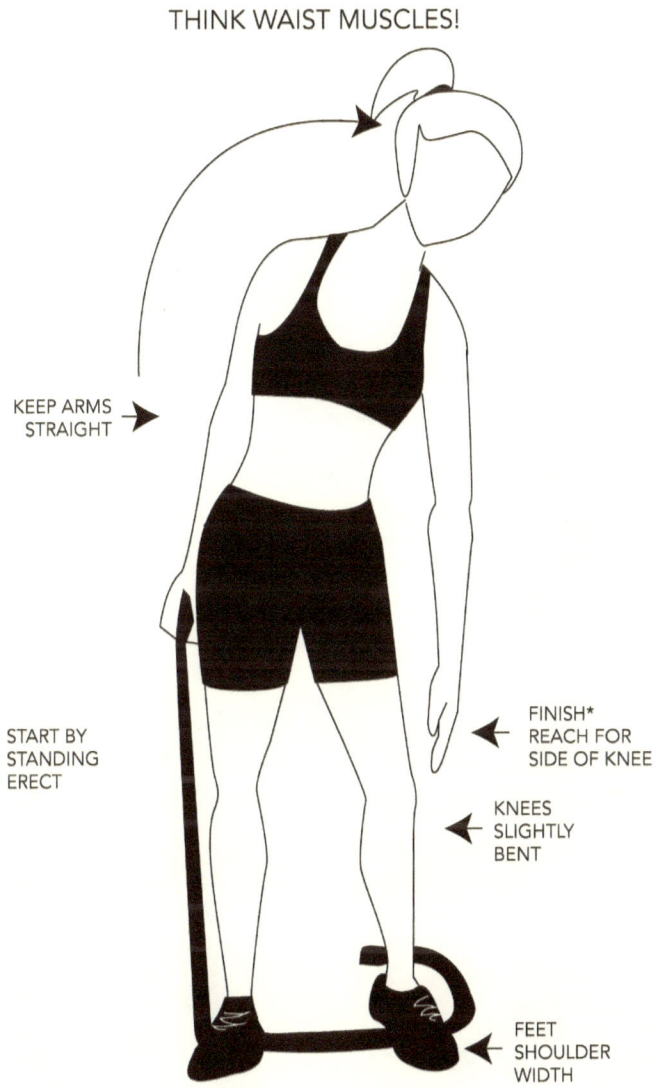

KEEP ARMS STRAIGHT

START BY STANDING ERECT

FINISH*
REACH FOR SIDE OF KNEE

KNEES SLIGHTLY BENT

FEET SHOULDER WIDTH

*REPEAT ON OTHER SIDE

Step on the band and grasp with your arms at your side. Bend side to side against the pull of the band to develop side core strength. This along with sit-ups will help with posture and core fitness.

Rear Shoulder

THINK UPPER BACK MUSCLES
AND REAR SHOULDER MUSCLES!

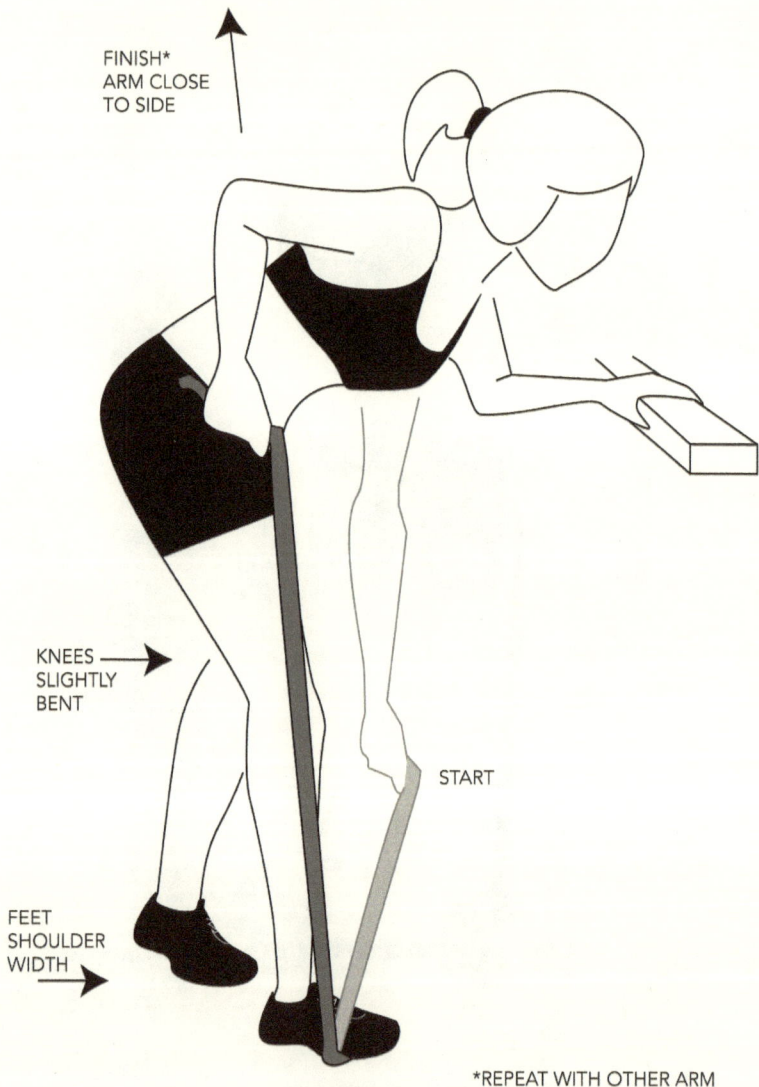

FINISH*
ARM CLOSE
TO SIDE

KNEES
SLIGHTLY
BENT

START

FEET
SHOULDER
WIDTH

*REPEAT WITH OTHER ARM

Place band under one foot with knees bent. Grasp band with same side hand and pull up. Change sides and repeat.

"Lats"

THINK UPPER BACK MUSCLES!

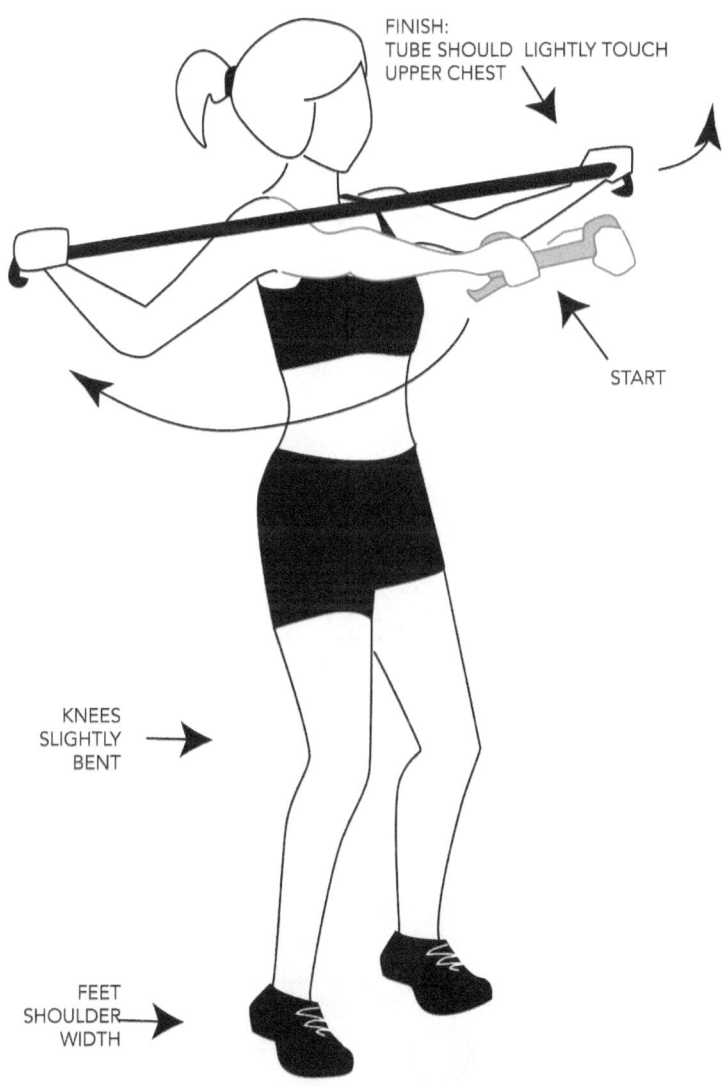

FINISH:
TUBE SHOULD LIGHTLY TOUCH
UPPER CHEST

START

KNEES
SLIGHTLY
BENT

FEET
SHOULDER
WIDTH

Grasp the band in front of you parallel to the floor and shoulder length apart. Now pull away and feel the muscles of your back contract. Release and repeat.

"Pecs"

THINK CHEST MUSCLES!

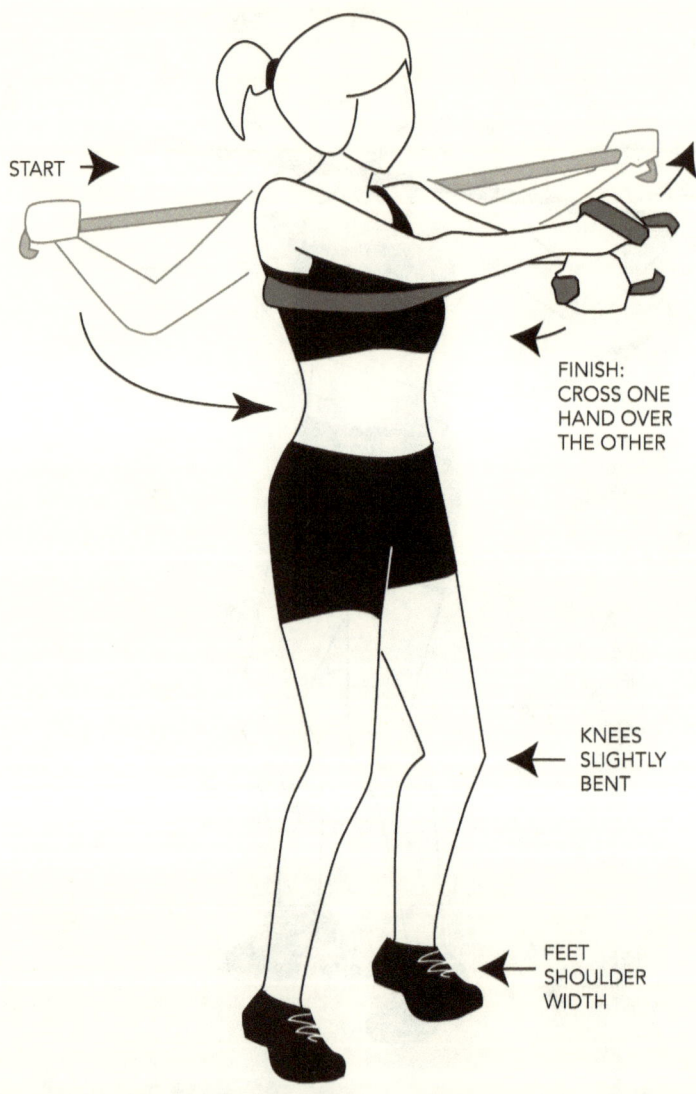

START ▶

FINISH:
CROSS ONE
HAND OVER
THE OTHER

KNEES
SLIGHTLY
BENT

FEET
SHOULDER
WIDTH

Place the band behind your back and push forward and across your body. This will contract the muscles of the chest.

If need be most of these exercises can be done one arm at a time. This reduces the tension on the band you are using. Once you can master 3 sets with both arms working together increase the band tension.

Next do sit-ups for 30 seconds. Lie on your back with knees slightly bent and hands grasped behind your head. Make sure elbows and arms are in line with the floor. Now flex your abdominal muscles and lift only a few inches off the floor and repeat. This is all the motion you need to work the core.

Finish the routine with push-ups for 30 seconds. Keep your back straight at all times as if in a plank position. If this is too difficult then do them with bent knees. This takes the stress off the shoulders and remains effective.

Now you have it: 10 resistance exercises and 10 aerobic intervals all completed between 10 and 20 minutes.

There are many more exercises that can be done with bands and they can be found on the internet. Do not become over enthusiastic. Master this program first and then when you are **ready,** advance.

For variation you can do all the band exercises as a complete set moving from one to the next in repetitions of 10 beginning with 30 seconds of jumping jacks and adding an aerobic motion for 30 -60 seconds including the sit-ups and push-ups before starting the cycle over. Try to work up to 3 sets of 10 repetitions with at least 30 – 60 seconds of interval aerobics.

SECTION III

SURGERY

7

Body Contouring: Skin Tightening
After Massive Weight Loss

It is my hope that early implementation of The Restore Point will help create healthy bodies and minds that need no surgical alterations. However, if your child was significantly overweight, there can be the additional burden of "the loose envelope" or sagging skin.

It is not possible to predict how a body's skin will shrink, even around a newly fit frame. Under these circumstances of very significant weight loss, body contouring surgery may be needed to complete the transformation.

> Although the need for body contouring is not always the result of a major weight loss, I feel I should address this all-too-common need. Whether by diet or bariatric surgery the body responds the same: stretched skin may not completely shrink back and the result is an unpredicted new set of circumstances that must be corrected.

Body contouring is the surgical process of eliminating excess skin and residual fat deposits after massive weight loss. A recent report published in the *Journal of Plastic and Reconstructive Surgery* tracked 100 patients, all of whom had dropped 100 pounds after bariatric surgery—the most extreme way of losing weight, and one which often leaves loose skin in its wake. Patients who did not deal with these skin issues gained back about 50 pounds on average. Patients who had had body contouring, in contrast, gained back only 13 pounds.

Once your child or teen has lost a significant amount of weight, he or she may find himself or herself dealing with excess skin—an issue which comes with its own complex series of challenges.

This is where the plastic surgeon's skill comes in.

Body contouring can help your child or teen feel and look "normal" after massive weight loss, but it is important to realize that "normal" after massive weight loss, and body contouring surgery, is not the same as a healthy normal child or teen's body that has always been at optimum weight.

If your exposure to the issue of body contouring surgery after weight loss is limited to what you may have seen on television reality shows, where the happy weight loss subject miraculously appears with tight skin and a gleaming smile, you may be shocked to hear what is really involved. A surgical solution is often necessary for the hanging skin that results from massive weight loss.

Body contouring is a complex issue where physical, emotional and financial considerations must all be considered.

Surgical improvements for the consequences of massive weight loss are available, and often necessary for complete restoration to whole, just like breast reconstruction is after mastectomy. But unlike breast reconstruction, post weight loss procedures are not always covered by insurance.

Safe and Sane Solutions First

In my first book, *The Safe and Sane Guide to Teenage Plastic Surgery (BenBella Books 2010)*, I outline the surgical, technical and financial considerations of body contouring. I also advise parents of kids and teens who are planning a major weight loss to look into costs and options for body contouring BEFORE the child or teen actually loses the weight.

Body contouring is again costly, and often not covered by insurance, so it is wise to assess the costs and payment options for this surgery before your child or teen hits his or her RESTORE POINT. If by good fortune your child does not need surgery you have a nest egg to put to other uses for your family – but at least you are prepared.

Tightening the Skin Envelope

Body contouring entails larger scars, more complex procedures, longer recoveries and bigger expenses than you may expect. Some of my patients—both kids and adults—have told me that taking off the weight initially was much easier than undergoing these procedures.

Surgeons call the largest organ of our bodies—the skin—an envelope. When a massive weight loss occurs, the skin envelope often remains at the size the former body weight initially stretched it into. This is where surgery comes in.

Questions to Ask When Considering Surgery

If body-contouring surgery is a possibility for your teen? Ask yourself the following questions.

1. **Has the weight loss been stable for at least one year?** This allows for nutritional stability and for the skin to shrink as much as possible. It also shows determination in keeping the weight off.
2. **Is my teen otherwise in good health?** Careful medical management is crucial to avoid surgical complications—particularly problems with wound healing.
3. **Does my teen smoke?** Nicotine hinders healing and must be eliminated from the system at least six weeks before surgery.
4. **Is my teen psychologically prepared for the surgeries and recovery?** This process can be arduous for patient and family.
5. **Do we all have realistic expectations?** Surgery will improve shape, but it cannot restore it to what it may have been without the weight gain.
6. **Are we prepared for the risks? Have we been informed?** All surgeries carry risks.

Teens or kids who need surgery on more than a single anatomic part are advised to find what is called a **Center of Excellence**. These centers are capable of staging and or stacking the multiple re-draping surgeries, which are often necessary to restore the body to a semblance of its original skin contour.

Risk vs. Reality

Before a discussion can be undertaken regarding body contouring surgical procedures, there must be time spent on the risks (this why prevention is the best remedy). Patients and their parents need to know that the procedures probably require a stay in the hospital, and may involve multiple surgeries (known as stages) over a few years. This should be discussed with the surgeon well in advance of the surgery so everyone understands, and is on board with the process.

Because of the significant amount of skin to be removed, body-contouring surgery poses greater risks than standard cosmetic procedures. The patient spends more time on the operating table, especially when the surgeon is working on more than one area of the body. Prolonged anesthesia can mean longer recovery time and an increased risk of deep vein thrombosis (DVT), a blood clot commonly in the legs that could cause pulmonary embolism and even death. To prevent such catastrophes, many centers are anti–coagulating (thinning the blood with medication) these types of patients. These treatments are state of the art, but carry their own risks of excess bleeding, bruising, and delays in wound healing. It is a delicate balance to optimize these individuals.

Since the removals of skin are frequently big, drains—tubes to carry away any fluid accumulations under the skin—are usually used and can remain for longer than in other cosmetic procedures. Large incisions also mean larger wounds to heal and longer scars than one may imagine.

Many surgeons place their patients in support garments for the post-operative recovery period. These help hold the tissues in place and provide support and security to the patients.

Most procedures require hospital stays of between one and four days. Multiple-site surgeries require multiple incisions and cause more discomfort. For this reason, many surgeons opt for staged procedures (one area at a time) over a few years. This allows patients to recover physically, emotionally, and financially.

The Types of Procedures by Body Part

Different areas of the body require different procedures. The farther you go down the body, the more significant the deformity and the more difficult it is to correct. Let's look at each area from the top of the body to the bottom.

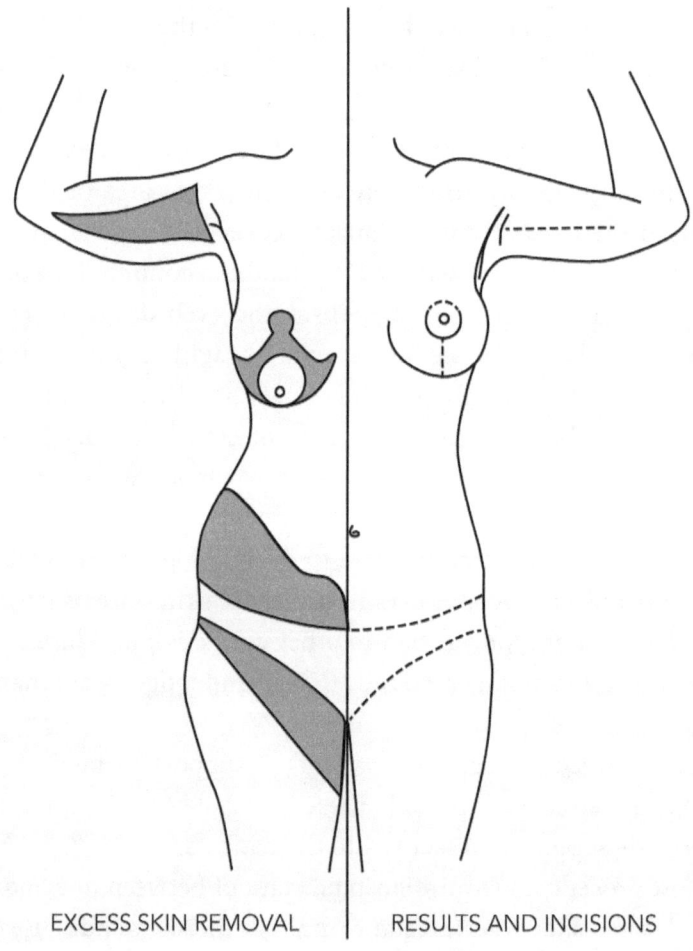

EXCESS SKIN REMOVAL   RESULTS AND INCISIONS

Face and Neck

Fortunately, even after significant weight loss, the face seems to be spared sagging. Face re-draping procedures in teens are rare. Occasionally, a neck liposuction may be needed (see the section on liposuction later in the chapter).

Breasts

Anything can happen with significant weight loss. It is possible for the breasts to reduce appropriately and become a non-issue. It is possible for them to shrink differently, resulting in size discrepancies. More often than not, the breasts sag and assume a much more elderly shape than a teen desires. Sagging breasts can be lifted. Sometimes the patient has lost so much weight that lifting is not enough and she also needs an augmentation. Occasionally, in spite of weight loss, the breasts remain disproportionately large and require a reduction. Thus, the patient may need a lift, a reduction, an augmentation, or a combination of these; so the procedures must be tailored to the situation.

In patients who have lost an extreme amount of weight, the excess skin can go beyond the breast edge onto the flank and back. The surgeon can perform an extended procedure to include this excess skin, but this procedure will increase the length of the scars.

Teen boys also can be faced with sagging breasts after weight loss and may require excisional surgeries as well to tighten the chest area and create a more masculine physique.

Arms

With loss of volume, upper-arm skin can sag. Although this is bothersome, it is often a lesser priority in the treatment plans of body contouring in teens. However, sometimes a teen has so much hanging skin on his or her arms—known as "bat wings"— the surgery becomes highly desirable. The surgery to fix this is called *brachioplasty* and it is done the same way on a teen, as it would be on an older individual. The procedure involves a long incision from the armpit (*axilla*) to the elbow. If the patient also has remaining excess fat, a spot liposuction may be added.

Abdomen

This is the most common area for correction in the teen weight-loss patient. When abdominal girth recedes, a hanging curtain of skin (*pannus*) can remain. This is very frustrating because it cannot be disguised the way breasts can be in custom bras. Bathing suits and light clothing are difficult to wear, and self-esteem diminishes. No matter how many crunches the patient does in the gym, the *pannus* remains. Oftentimes, a patient and family will seek consultation, thinking that a minimal-scar liposuction will make it disappear. But only excision of the skin will resolve the problem.

There are two forms of excisional surgery for the surgeon and patient to consider for this situation: ***panniculectomy*** and ***abdominoplasty***. In both procedures, the incision is large and extends from hip to hip across the front of the abdomen along the panty line. The goal is to redrape the front of the torso and, if needed, lift a sagging *mons pubis* (pubic area) as well.

Panniculectomy removes the hanging curtain of skin, but it does nothing for the upper abdomen. It is a very useful procedure that can bring both cosmetic and functional relief from the rashes and irritations that often occur when the abdominal skin rubs against the pubic skin. Insurance companies will consider this for reimbursement if the patient can show documentation of dermatological problems (***intertrigonal infections***) in the pannus folds. The procedure is a direct excision of the curtain and involves no undermining (radical elevations) of skin. Healing is usually straightforward, and the complications are few. Panniculectomy helps to boost self-esteem and is a great first start for patients requiring multiple procedures.

Abdominoplasty is a "panniculectomy plus" procedure. The skin is pulled away up to the lower rib edges. The exposed abdominal muscles can then be tightened with sutures. Next, the skin is pulled down and the excess (the skin that hangs below the incision line) removed. The belly button is repositioned to a more youthful position as the skin curtain is resected.

Drains are used in both procedures, and both surgeries take between two and four hours under general anesthesia. Patients usually remain in the hospital for one day.

Liposuction may be used on the flank regions following the resections to smooth out the edges.

In some situations, the patient has lost so much weight that the horizontal incision is not enough and an up-and-down incision must be added. This "fleur-de-lis" pattern allows for even more skin to be removed, but it also adds a significant vertical scar that is hard to hide.

Thighs

As we move down the body, the severity of the sagging increases. Many weight-loss patients—despite hours of aerobics—suffer from loose skin on the inner thighs. This can be unattractive, and it also causes discomfort from continual rubbing.

A medial thigh lift removes the excess skin of the upper inner thigh. Incision patterns vary based on the deformity. Sometimes they are restricted to the groin creases, but other cases require an additional incision down the inside of the thigh from the groin to the knee.

Body Lifts

Some patients are physically, emotionally, and financially able to undergo multiple contouring procedures in one operation. These combinations are called body lifts.

Lower Body Lift

The lower body lift procedure is more than an extended abdomino-plasty or panniculectomy. Here the patient is turned over and the buttocks and thighs are lifted as well. It involves more time than abdominoplasty or panniculectomy alone, and the potential for complications increases as more is done. Recovery is also more arduous because a lower-body lift hinders walking and sitting in the very early recovery phase.

Upper Body Lift

An upper-body lift, which is a set of procedures, corrects the breasts and arms, and extends onto the upper back to remove the rolls of excess skin there as well. Like the lower-body lift, this combination procedure takes longer and is more stressful for the patient in recovery than a single procedure.

Excisional body-contouring procedures can be very helpful to teens who feel miserable and trapped in their own skin after massive weight loss. The price is high in both cost and risks, but the rewards can be great. It is critical that a patient understands that incisions and scars are extensive, and although they will fade they are permanent. Body-contouring surgery is not a quick fix, except in cases in which weight losses have resulted in singular but real deformities. These can often be handled singularly by one of the above individual procedures.

Liposuction

One of the reasons for the liposuction's popularity is the minimal incision aspect. However, this can be misleading. Although the access sites are small, the spaces created to remove the fat are large. Furthermore, the smaller incisions do not mean fewer risks.

Liposuction should only be done on teens who have met the strictest of criteria. Many teens believe this to be the ideal quick-fix procedure with basically no incisions, and they may seek it as an easy weight-loss method. The surgeon and parents should make sure the teen is mature enough to understand that liposuction is surgery with risks.

I will consider liposuction alone when isolated deposits of fat remain after a teen has normalized his/her body weight with a healthy diet and exercise program. Patients most often request my services for the outer thighs (the so-called "riding britches deformity") and under the neck. These are simple surgeries with rapid recoveries. Liposuction can also be used to supplement the excisional body-contouring methodologies described above when an area needs further refinement.

Prevention

As you read through these lists of procedures you can see why I am passionate about prevention—saving teens from having to undergo these surgeries.

Although all of these surgeries are often extremely successful, it is important to understand the time, cost and risks involved.

It is also important to understand that although we can come close to making the body appear normal after massive weight loss it is never as if the problem never occurred.

Prevention, prevention, prevention is the key.

A gradual weight loss of a moderate amount of weight on a child or teen may help the skin envelope regain its original contours but a consistently healthy weight from day one is the best way to avoid this major challenge in a kid or teen's life.

Afterword

Restore, Refresh, Renew Daily

It has been a long personal journey and commitment of mine to try and bring forth principles that can be separated from hype and fad. Interestingly, public recognition of child and teen weight issues has finally caught up with what I have known for a long time – we are at a generational health crisis. In fact, this manuscript was originally drafted 15 years ago and rejected … "as there was no market for a book on the subject of teenage obesity."

As you turn the final pages, remind yourself of principles – guideposts on an evolutionary journey for continued survival and well-being.

Facts Not Fads

There is a lot of talk about the need to live a new/old "Paleo" inspired lifestyle. A New York Times feature lauded the advent of "Saber-tooth Moms" who skip science fairs to play in muddy creeks or wander through the woods with their Paleo-brought-up-broods and who wouldn't dream of sending their kids to school without a lunchbox full of Paleo brownies.

I want to stress that that kind of lifestyle is NOT necessary for families that want their kids to stay at their new RESTORE POINT.

My program is based on nutritional principles I have personally seen work in obese kids and teens (and adults).

Eating this way does not require you to fit your bedroom out like a cave, wear amber goggles when watching TV at night, or snack on slabs of meat, rather than on food that tastes like food.

Connecting your body's new rhythms to your brain—in essence "re-wiring" your behavioral circuits to live the RESTORE POINT and the FOOD WHEEL are about MAKING THIS PROGRAM PART OF YOUR DAILY LIFE. This is the exact opposite of following a fad.

This is why I have deliberately not included menus or provided ways to mimic processed foods but rather, have suggested ways for you to teach your kids to "forage" for nutritionally sound food choices out in the real life big, bad world of "Fast Food," "Chips," and "10-ounce sugared sodas."

What I *am* recommending in this simple, principle-based system is that the mind *listen* once again to the body's instinctual programming, so that mind and body are working together for our health and well being.

All lifestyle changes require constant work to maintain and not slip back into old emotionally- friendly habits.

Some individuals may require counseling by nutritionists, therapists, trainers – all serving as "coaches" and "cheerleaders" to keep your teen on the correct path of good health for life.

Do not be afraid to embrace help when needed. They are not crutches – they are support systems. Left alone many will slip back.

Do As I Do Not As I Say

One of the best ways to anchor the changes in this book in your child or teen's life is to practice them yourself.

When a child or teen sees his or her parent enacting the changes that are being proposed for him, lifestyle shifts stick.

The reason I stress the Restore Point as a series of principles is that these are a *constant*—they will always keep you and your family on track for a fit and healthy life. But in order to keep that system consistently well maintained, vigilance is needed.

Think of it this way—once you've restored your computer to an earlier, working program point, you would not turn around and download some new malware to clog its memory again would you?

Keeping a computer free of viruses and malware is an ongoing process.

The Restore Point Weekly Virus Scan

Ask yourself and your kids these questions at some point every week:

1. Am I feeling energetic and healthy or slow and lethargic? Do I need to adjust my protein levels? Do I need to take in more food, or eat less?
2. Am I getting enough sleep?
3. Have I allowed non-Restore Point-Program foods into my weekly diet? How are they affecting me?
4. Have I been moving and getting outdoors enough? Am I getting some activity every day?
5. Have I been overdoing my active life?
6. Are processed foods creeping back into my diet?
7. Am I taking the time to really enjoy what I eat?
8. Have I substituted juice for food on too many occasions this week?
9. Am I drinking enough water?

Once you and your family have gotten to your own personal RESTORE POINTS, consider a weekly VIRUS SCAN the way you'd run a vigilance program on your computer.

There is too often a tendency to fall prey to the "Madison Avenue" promotions of "6 weeks to this or 12 weeks to that."

Stay the course and remain steadfast to the principles that we have evolved to and have guided us to be here today. It was, and is, how we are programmed. It is all about balance, keeping your cultural software compatible with your genetic operating system.

Now that you have reached the end of this book, realize that it is only the beginning to a reset in your thinking about food and movement. Adhering and applying the outlined principles will make you and your child feel and look better. And when you look and feel better, you are better!

Works Consulted

Atkins, R. 1981. *Dr. Atkins Diet Revolution*, Bantam

Beson, P. 1971, Cecil-Loeb Textbook of Medicine, W.B Saunders Company

Booher, J.M. 1925, *Scientific Weight Control*, Continental Scale Works

Cash, T. ed. et al, 2004, *Body Image: Theory, Research and Clinical Practice*, Guilford Press

Eaton, S. 1988, *The Paleolithic Prescription*, Harper & Row

Kolata, G. 2007, *Rethinking Thin*, Farrar & Straus & Giroux

Lopez, R. 2002, *Teen Health Book*, W.H. Norton & Company

Lukash, F. 2010, *The Safe and Sane Guide to Teenage Plastic Surgery*, BenBella

Ogeda, A., ed. 2003, *Body Image-Teen Decisions*, Greenhaven Press

Rimm, S., 2004, *Rescuing the Emotional Lives of Overweight Children*, Rodale

Stein, L. 1988, *Bloomingdales Eat Healthy Diet*, St. Martin's Press

Steward, H., 1995, *Sugar Busters*, Ballantine Press

Thiessen, D. 1998, *Survival of the Fittest*, Morgan Press

Watnik, H. 1985, *Exer-Stretch*

About the Author

FREDERICK N. LUKASH, MD, FACS, FAAP has consistently been voted one of "Americas Top Doctors" by the Castle Connolly guide and by the Consumers' Research Council of America. Dr. Lukash is a board-certified cosmetic and reconstructive plastic surgeon, specializing in pediatric and adolescent body image issues. In practice in New York City and Long Island since 1981, he is an assistant clinical professor of surgery at the Albert Einstein College of Medicine and the Hofstra University School of Medicine. He is a fellow in the American College of Surgeons and the American Academy of Pediatrics.

Dr. Lukash is a member of all the major plastic surgical societies—the American Society for Aesthetic Plastic Surgery, the American Association of Plastic Surgeons, the American Association of Pediatric Plastic Surgeons, the American Society of Maxillofacial Surgeons, and the American Society of Plastic Surgeons, for which he is a media spokesperson on the topic of teens and plastic surgery. He has also been involved with the Plastic Surgery Research Council, the American Cleft Palate-Craniofacial Association, Operation Smile and Surgical Aid to the Children of the World.

Dr. Lukash's previous book, *The Safe and Sane Guide to Teenage Plastic Surgery* (BenBella, 2010) is a watershed book in its field and one that drew praise from both the medical profession and the media. He has written many articles and textbook content for the academic plastic surgical community, including a position paper on plastic surgery teenagers for the American Society of Plastic Surgeons.

Dr. Lukash received his college and medical degrees from Tulane University. His postgraduate training in surgery and plastic surgery includes Emory University, State University of New York, and Harvard University, where he has held the position of Instructor in Surgery.

In the media, Dr. Lukash has been featured as a speaker on teens and health for CNN, *GoodDay New York, The Today Show* and many others.

Visit www.drlukash.com and www.therestorepoint.com for updates and blogs on the topics of teens, health, obesity and body image.